Praise for Caitlin
OF MATE

"Eye-opening stories told with true passion."
-*Kailey Esser, Registered Midwife,*
College of Midwives of Ontario

"Caitlin Arlene, a sensitive and charismatic investigator on the maternal health issue, conveys an unmissable sense of compassion through her writing. She relays Malawians' testimonies with dignity and care, while prompting the reader to wonder: what can I do?

Hard facts and statistics, cushioned by Caitlin's thoughtful narrative, evoke a feeling of unrest in the reader. Why is it acceptable for women to give birth on the side of the road, in the dead of night? Why is the high maternal and infant mortality rate so widely tolerated? Mama leaves the audience shaking from the injustices too many women and their babies encounter daily.

Read *Mama* and you'll open the door to a nation and its people, whose passionate resilience in curing the maternal health epidemic overrides the dark reality that enfolds Malawi every day."
-*Syndey Hildebrandt, Journalist,*
TimesWPG

MAMA

TRUE STORIES
OF MATERNAL HEALTH
IN MALAWI

CAITLIN ARLENE

atmosphere press

© 2021 Caitlin Arlene

Published by Atmosphere Press

Cover design by Ronaldo Alves

No part of this book may be reproduced without permission from the author except in brief quotations and in reviews.

atmospherepress.com

May your eyes be open and your hearts be broken.

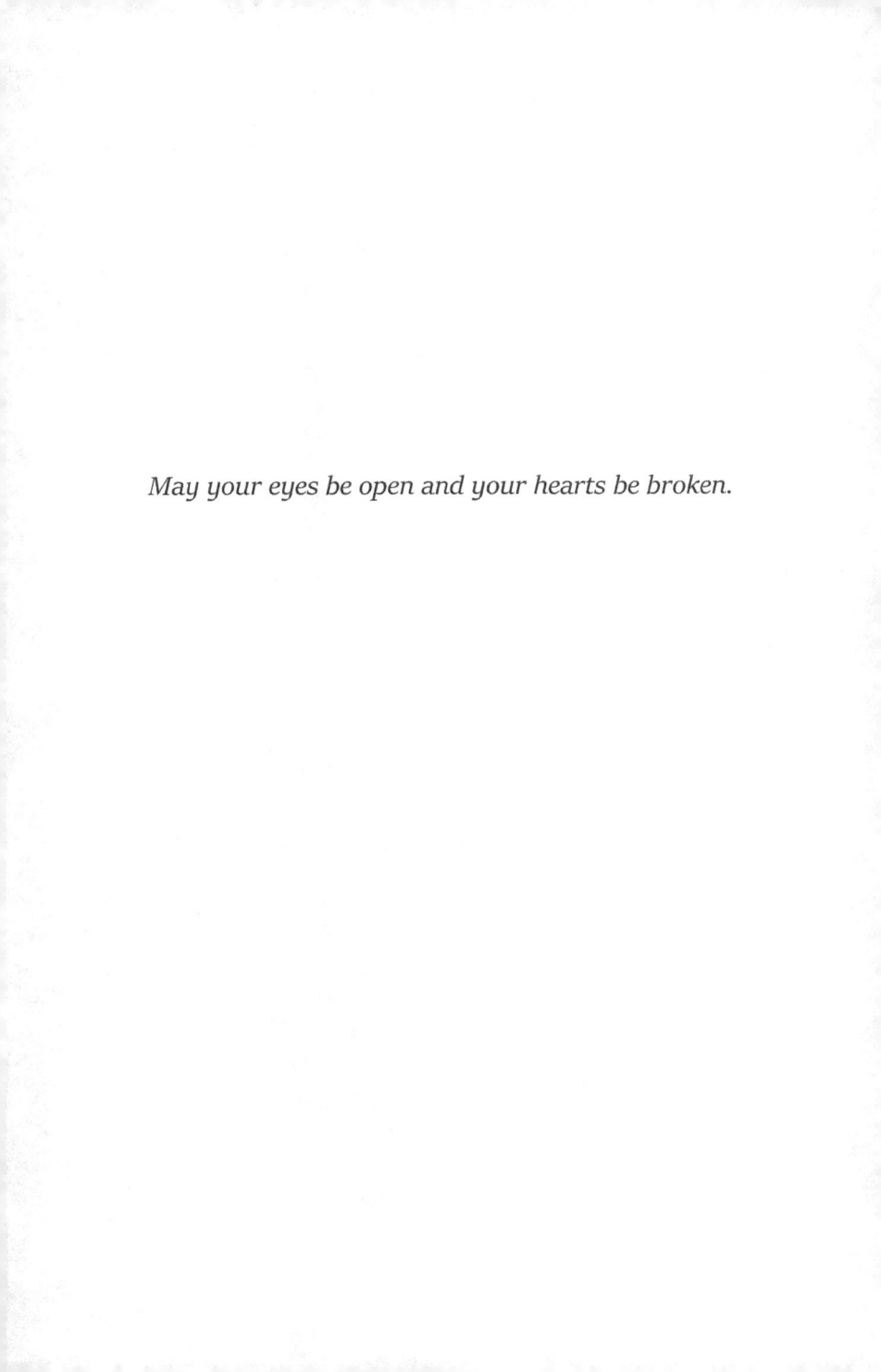

TABLE OF CONTENTS

TO BEGIN	3
BIMBI HEALTH FACILITY	9
AGNESS	15
AARON	21
FRANCIS	29
MIRIAM, PARTIMA, BACHALO	35
GLADYS	43
KILATU	51
MRS. MVULA	59
FYNES	65
MARIA	71
KATHERINE	77
MR. + MRS. MCHENGA	83
DYSON + ESNAT	91
GERTRUDE	99
DECEMBER	105
KEVIN	111
CHARLES #1 + CHARLES #2	119
THE END	127

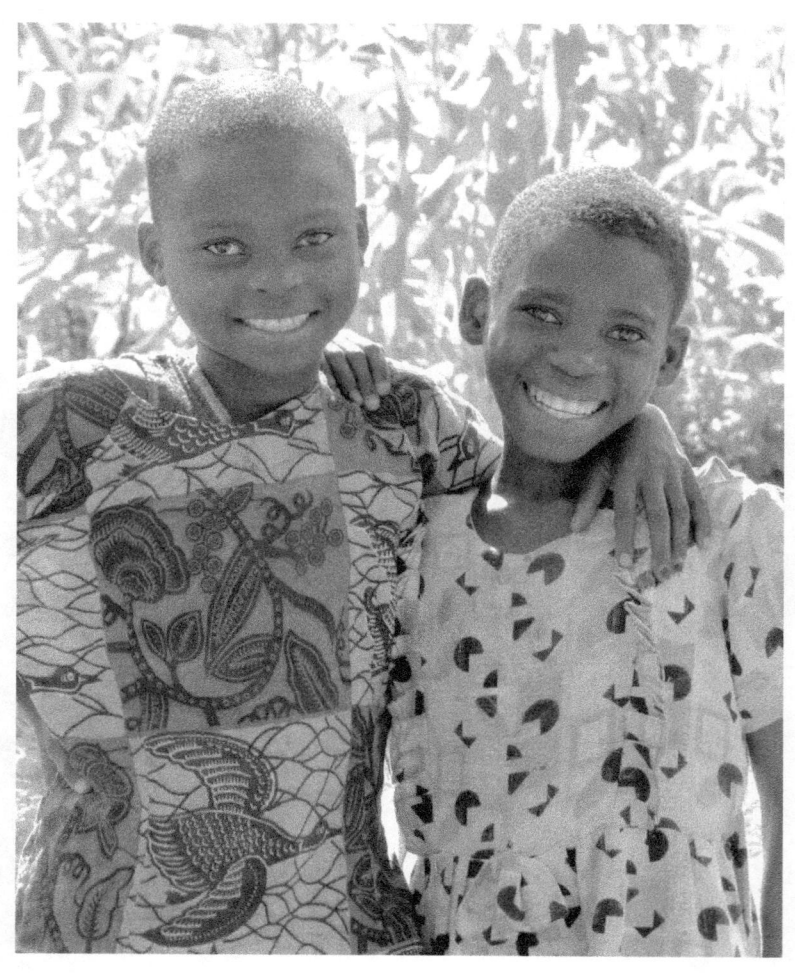

TO BEGIN

I've felt apprehension every time I've taken this pen to the paper. A hundred first sentences have scrawled through my mind—a hundred perfect words and paragraphs to commence this story. But I haven't had the courage to make them certain until now.

It's not the story itself that causes me fear but the daunting task of doing it justice. I look at the many mothers, children, families, midwives and nurses who each carry an equivalent and fascinating story. I'm humbled by their confidence and intimidated by the messages they've passed on to me. My loyalty to these compelling pieces of their lives begs me forward, yet each time I close my eyes and return to their homes, remembering the creases in their faces or the tone of their voices, I can't help but shake under the gravity of their stories. How can my simple words capture the magnitude of their experiences? How can I adequately manipulate the English alphabet to portray the lives of those whose voices spoke to me in a different language entirely?

It's important to emphasize the reality of the contents of this book. The testimony I share here is a compilation of true stories—all the words herein are inspired by the very women, children, and men that I've spoken to. Every one of these people laugh and cry, live and love in the same way that anyone else does. And as it is with all strangers and newfound friends, we've peeped through the keyhole into one room of their complex lives and built conclusions from the jagged scene within. I'd like to think that this little glimpse, albeit a tiny piece of their puzzle, offers a new perspective and a promise of a clearer image of who these beautiful strangers are, the nature of their struggle, and the hope mixed with their pain.

These reasons alone explain why I write with a trembling hand. To demonstrate their lives, largely juxtapositions of my own, in a way that is true and honorable to them and their culture will not be an easy task. This mission, to bring to life the stories through which I only see from the outside is not simple. But here I am, called forward by the necessity for the proclamation of their stories.

Over the past several years, the issue of maternal health in Africa has weighed heavy on my heart. I was first introduced to the cause while researching an article for a mission's organization called Emmanuel International, where I worked for several years as a summer student. At that time, they had just begun a maternal health project, and my job was to write the introductory article to send to their donors. Their particular program was called PROMISE.[*]

PROMISE was an urgent and successful program

---

[*] PROMISE stands for **Pro**moting **M**aternal, Newborn, **I**nfant and Child **S**ustainable Health **E**fforts. The program is a consortium of three Canadian charities whose purpose is to reduce maternal and child mortality in developing countries. Children Believe established their efforts in Ghana; the Adventist Development and Relief Agency (ADRA) took the mission to Rwanda; and Emmanuel International Canada (EIC) rooted PROMISE in Malawi, from where the stories of this book emerge.

whose mission was to reduce maternal and child mortality throughout three African nations: Ghana, Rwanda, and Malawi. Founded by three Canadian charities, they were funded by international donors whose contributions were then matched seven-fold by the Government of Canada.

As I researched deeper into the maternal health crisis, my heart flooded. Sympathy, surprise, unease, and motivation pushed me forward in a way that disquieted myself. The cause was necessary, the issues were imminent, and the urgency was validated.

Close to 830 women worldwide die every single day due to preventable complications throughout pregnancy and childbirth.[i] Of that 830 women, 99% of them live in a developing nation. In 2015, 2.7 million babies died within days of their birth; an equal amount were recorded as stillborn. Their heartbreaking deaths are results of multiple causes, including infections, disease, blood pressure, and complications during childbirth. Distance, poor infrastructure, and lack of education within these developing nations also influence women not to seek proper care when such issues occur.

For so long, this issue has gone unnoticed—unattended to by governments and caretakers and organizations. It wasn't until the turn of the century that the mothers were finally noticed by the world. In September 2000, 191 of the United Nations member states signed a declaration committing them to eight specific developmental goals as the new millennium began. The fourth and fifth of these Millennium Developmental Goals (MDGs)[ii] were to reduce child mortality and to improve maternal health. As such, the entire world has watched as our leaders prioritized and addressed the very topics that these pages highlight.

The mournful reality of poor maternal health culture is manifested in heartbreak and loss of life. Shortage of wholesome nourishment prevails, often leading to disease, malnutrition, and premature passing. Lack of infrastructure means millions have limited access to health facilities, often giving birth without the assistance of any trained caretaker—a doctor, midwife, or otherwise. Even simple complications in pregnancy can be the highest risk for a mother and her child; often a mere hiccup can go unattended for too long with irreversible consequences. So many mothers have lost their children. So many children have lost their mothers.

When I uncovered the troubling numbers as a young summer student, I was momentarily consumed by a feeling of helplessness. My thoughts spun with concern, "What if this reality applied to someone I love? How would I respond if I knew the individual behind the statistics?"

It was in those moments that I determined the need for this very book. I pledged allegiance to the 830 nameless faces that die each day, compelled by the desire to know them and make their stories known. I spent the next two years building on my idea; reaching out to various contacts, writing proposals, and following up on introductions. Finally, a providential door opened, and I leaped through it. Unfunded, unsponsored, and propelled solely by my passion for the untold stories herein, I flew forward to fulfill my promise to the testimonies I pursued.

I landed with the program into the warm heart of Africa, speaking to every person I came into contact with, collecting all the stories that I could find. I was privileged to see, experience, and put to words the hope that is being provided. This program and many like it are emerging throughout the continent offering culture-shifting services, training, and instruction.

My hands tremble no more—my fear is gone. With every letter that slips into this collection, my devotion to these stories increases. These stories must be heard. For the sake of the mothers and children and families in Malawi and across the world.

Dear reader, this book is for you. You may do with it what you will, but my prayer is for your eyes to be opened wide to the realities the humans in these stories must face, and that you have the comfort never to endure it yourself. My prayer is that your heart will be broken for the maternal health crisis, and you will somehow be stirred to action. And if no understanding has been instilled, and no awakening has been had; if my mission has all but failed, then I implore you to take the time and come see for yourself the hurting and the hope.

Come and see the cliffs that have been conquered and the mountains to be climbed.

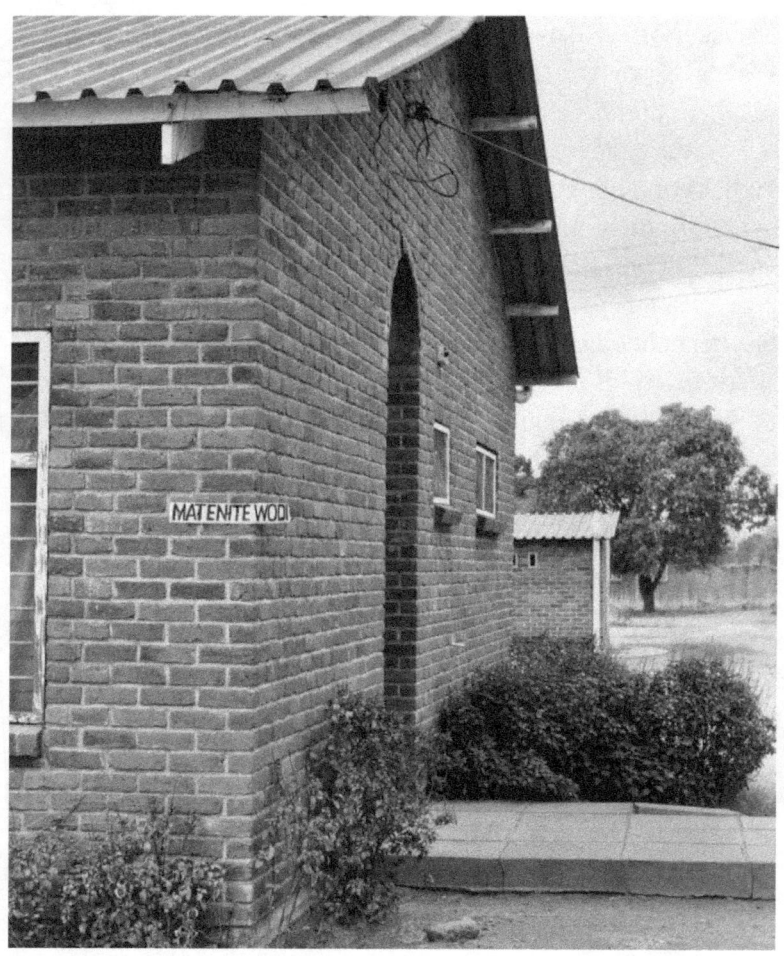

BIMBI HEALTH FACILITY

It took us just under an hour to reach the facility. It would have taken us a little longer if it were a different time of year, but Malawi was in the height of their dry season, and it had been months since the rains attacked the roads with potholes and thick mud. Instead, only the deepest craters remained, baked deep into the red clay roads. Similarly, there were fewer people on the roads than there might have previously been when the air was cooler. Whether that can be attributed to the time of day or season of the year, it is much harder to tell. I could, however, comfortably conclude that the dry, dusty heat and undeterred sun was enough to dissuade anyone from moving very far about.

Needless to say, our bumpy back-roads journey didn't take us as long as it *could* have, and for that, I was very thankful.[*]

The Bimbi Health Facility was not as I imagined it

---

[*] The last time I journeyed through the Malawian fields was just after their rainy season a few years before. The roads were at their most decrepit state, and though the drivers were skilled and experienced at maneuvering the vehicle around the craters, I was still left with bruised legs and knees from all the jostling about. I'll never complain about any journey or adventure I take, but I will confess that those rides were among the least comfortable ones I took.

would be. The picture I conjured in my mind was based on a Malawian hospital I had visited a few years ago during my first expedition to the country. Though the image in my head did not match reality, it was neither better nor worse, more rugged or modern. It was simply different. I learned long ago not to hold on to expectations, and I've rarely been disappointed by anything since.

The facility carried two open concept waiting rooms, with neither doors nor walls to separate the wooden benches from the outside. There were two lamp-less hallways to either side of the waiting areas with about three or four offices and care rooms down each. What walls the facility did have were made of clay bricks, rising high to a tin roof. The offices themselves were modest, with sun-faded white paint that had been chipped from years of weather.

Covering the various patchy locations on the walls were an assortment of posters. Eye charts, doctors' notes, hand-washing instructions—all printed on the same thin sheets of printer paper. They were posted at eye level in various locations across the room. I could only understand the use of a handful of the posters, as the majority of them were written with the rolling vowels and constants of the Chichewa language.

The Bimbi Health Facility is one of hundreds located throughout the country. The District of Zomba is parent to this particular facility and oversees thirty-two sister clinics in the large area. The Malawian health care system, though complicated by many factors such as poor infrastructure, lack of resources and supplies, medical practitioners, and overall funding, is actually less complex than I first expected to see.

First comes the Malawian Ministry of Health, which oversees the education of medicine, the establishment of medical practices, and helps provide funding to the districts throughout the country.[iii] From there, medical care is slowly broken down by district, communities, and then individual villages.

For instance, Zomba is one of twenty-eight districts in Malawi. Each district has a centralized hospital with offices that oversee the health care distribution across the district. Some districts may be home to several hospitals, depending on various contributing factors such as population, infrastructure, and income. At this level, it's possible to see privatized hospitals which are often funded by churches, organizations, and other outside sources. These hospitals aren't funded by the Malawian government but are generally supported and accommodated by them in any case.

Each district oversees a number of health clinics and facilities within their borders. The Bimbi Health Facility is one of such locations, and all of its programs, workers, and resources are allocated by the Zomba District Health Facility. These community clinics are dispersed throughout the district according to population, need, and location.

Our particular building of interest, Bimbi Health Facility, serves as a center for all the surrounding villages. Even though these facilities are placed in the most optimal locations between villages, it still may take a patient several hours to arrive, particularly if they have no quick mode of transportation or must travel by foot.

Each health facility is composed of a team of health administrators who each have various levels of training.

Because there is such a shortage of educated doctors, the patients who attend these facilities are primarily treated by a nurse or other similar assistant. In every case, however, the role of the Health Surveillance Assistant (HSA) is fulfilled.

The HSA is the individual dispatched from the centralized health facility who travels from village to village, ensuring proper health measures are being met within the communities. Because many of these communities are so remotely located, it's often easier for the HSA to travel the distance and dust-covered roads bringing health assistance to the villages, instead of waiting for the villages to come to them.

At the same time, the HSA is also able to deliver any special instructions or replace the depleted supplies to the final piece of the Malawian health care puzzle. Village clinics—often no more complicated than a pantry-sized storeroom—serve as the most local place where villagers can come to receive any prescribed medication or similar services. More often than not, these clinics primarily carry malaria medication, HIV and AIDS prescriptions, and very basic supplements. The volunteers who take care of these clinics are community leaders who will often take on the responsibility to travel door-to-door, encouraging their community to maintain the health practices they have been taught over the years.

My first steps into the open waiting room were observed by nearly sixty pairs of eyes. The benches were full and overflowing with the yellows, oranges, blues, and greens of the jubilant Malawian dress. Mothers and children of all ages were crowding the room, spilling out into the yard with colorful patience. Every five minutes or so, the office door would drift open, and out would sweep the bright pattern of the previous patient. Next in line would catch the door before it was even fully exited and squeeze herself or her child through the frame. The metal fastener would click shut, one rainbow would disappear and the other would leave, and one would take their spot in line.

If I had closed my eyes and transported myself back to the office of my family doctor in Canada, I could not have imagined a greater contrast. For the few times that I've ever had to wait in a clinic, office or even emergency room, I never once had to sit on the floor or outside of the building because the benches had reached capacity. Canadians sometimes complain about the long wait time, but I've never been fortieth in line since 5 a.m. for an undetermined ailment without a promise of treatment. I've never questioned that the air I was breathing was anything less than over-sanitized, confirmed by the ever-present aroma of rubbing alcohol and hand sanitizer.

But this time I stood and watched the door re-open, my nose dulled by the dust carried through the wall-less room. Brushing shoulders with the woman next to me, I wondered what I ever could have complained about before.

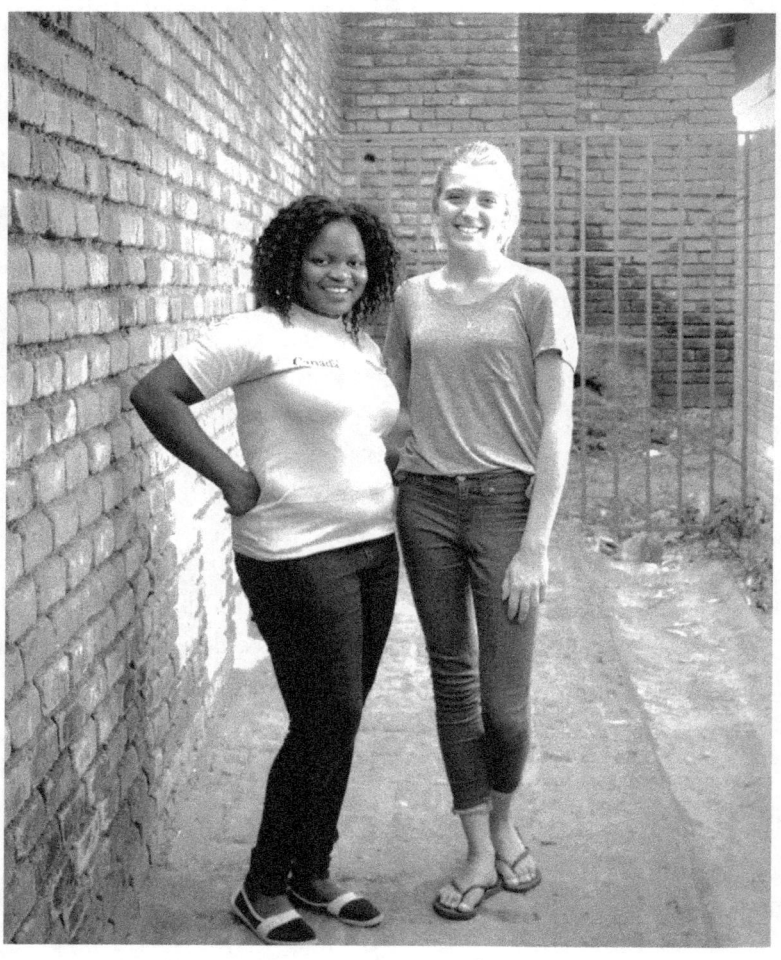

AGNESS

The words written within these pages are owed to many people. To those willing to offer a piece of themselves to be in it. To those who helped facilitate my lodging, made themselves available for my many questions and queries. But one woman must be introduced, for she became my immediate companion and constant treasure throughout the journey.

Agness.

We met the very afternoon that I landed in Malawi, after my generous hosts gave me a few hours to settle into my temporary home and notify my family that I had arrived safely. The home I was staying in doubled as the Malawian headquarters to the organization that put on the very project I would be following over the next several weeks. Aside from the short hallway that separated the sleeping quarters from the rest of the building, the rooms were host to a constant flow of foot traffic, project meetings, Bible studies, and employees and volunteers.

There was a separate brick building two steps downhill and a sturdy retaining wall away where groups of field staff would gather and disperse throughout the day, collectively attending to their various projects and missions. It was here that I first met Agness and the rest of the PROMISE administration.

After unpacking and recovering from the long, air-sick plane ride, I made my way down the red stone path to the PROMISE office. Having worked in Malawi and with various translators before, I had come prepared with a few expectations, and prepared myself accordingly—but the moment that I met Agness, I knew I could proceed with full confidence.

Agness is the kind of woman who excels at anything she dedicates herself to. From the ever-ready smile on her lips to the friendly bounce of her braided hair, she became a fast friend. Not only was she an administrator and community facilitator to the Maternal Health Project, she was incredibly insightful and keen to understand the goals I had outlined for my research. Agness arranged every meeting, every transport, and every event that I would be attending while in the field.

Also acting as an English-Chichewa teacher in the nearby city every weekend, Agness would patiently laugh with me as I struggled through the various Chichewa phrases I practiced while our heads bobbed up and down with the untamed roads in the Malawian bush.

I hadn't even prayed for a companion who would be as important and valuable as Agness would become, but as every day passed, I could only express my increasing gratitude for her presence.

One early morning as our team set out down the long journey to our community of the day, Agness requested that we make a quick stop at her house, which was on the way. Our large truck jostled left, bouncing down a sleepy market street until we arrived at a small concrete house. It was painted a faded turquoise on its bottom half, contrasted by a stark white plaster that reached to the tin roof.

"I'll be right back," She called to us waiting in the truck as she ducked under a drying *chitenge*[*] on the clothesline and toward an open door.

A few minutes and curious neighbors passed by before Agness emerged again, having retrieved whatever it was she had forgotten to bring along that morning. On her hip was a tiny version of herself: a two-year-old daughter who already carried the same inquiring joy of her mother.

"She wanted to say hello to you before we leave!" Agness explained, laughing as her lookalike suddenly hid her face. "Go on, say hello!" She prodded.

Agness's little girl was adorned with obvious love, accessorising with pink beads in her hair and a short necklace. Bulky letters were patterned between the beads of her necklace, spelling out her name, Hosannah.

Hosannah is a liturgical exclamation in Christianity, one of praise, triumph, and thankfulness. Hosannah was also the most fitting name for a child of Agness.

After greeting her, I smiled as I watched the young girl tread back to her yard and Agness stepped back into the truck. 'Hosannah' would be my own stream of praise and thankfulness as I continued to work with my brilliant translator and guide. 'Hosannah' would be my thoughts on every sunset drive back to our home base—filled with the heavy stories collected and gratefulness that I could carry them with me at all.

"Hosannah!" I would think, each time I watched Agness translate my questions and relay their responses.

---

[*] A *chitenge* is the most versatile fabric in the country. Towel-sized and lightweight, they're used as skirts, wraps, dresses, baby slings, floormats, curtains, and more. They often come in the brightest patterns and lively colors.

'Hosannah' would be my thoughts as she offered freely her own understanding and expertise, not just relaying a translation, but what it meant culturally and individually.

"Hosannah!" I whisper to myself now as I reflect on the blessing Agness is, not only to this very book, but to the entire world she touches.

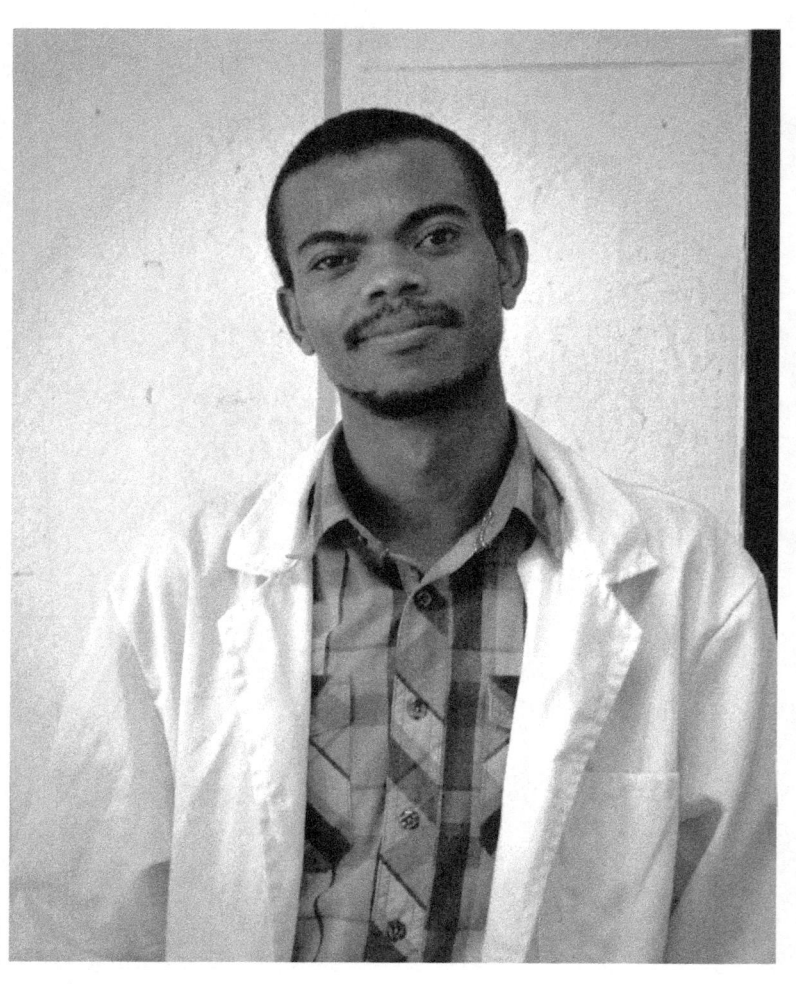

AARON

"We are going in now," Agness said to me, starting towards the door. A woman exited, carrying a child whose heaving sobs had quieted by exhaustion. The mother grabbed a corner of her time-worn *chitenge* to clear the shine that glistened on the skin between the child's nose and mouth.

"Come, it is our time," She called to me again, catching the door and holding it open for me. We were headed into the only active community clinic within Bimbi's facility reach.

"I'm sorry!" I murmured to the woman who I had to pass to enter. I looked down, but not soon enough to avoid the gaze of all the patients who were still waiting their turn. I wanted to call out, "I'm sorry! I'm not butting in line! I just have a few questions I want to ask him!" But I knew that they knew I wasn't a patient that just didn't want to wait my turn. If my camera and notebook weren't enough to give it away, it would have been the color of my skin.

A blonde-haired, blue-eyed *mzungu*[*] is a notable appearance in this area. Communities here are very close-knit, so they would have known me if I were local. In the same breath, the community surrounding the Bimbi Health Facility has often been a popular area for humanitarian organizations, and so the people would be used to seeing a few *azungu* and representatives of those organizations popping into their facilities. Though I felt the guilt of making them wait just a little longer, I saw in their gaze a tired understanding, and it was enough to encourage me into the room.

"*Muli bwanji*," a curious voice called out the custom Chichewa greeting. He continued in English, "Hello, you are welcomed!"

The owner of the greeting was Aaron, a medical assistant and the one in charge of the entire facility. Aaron studied in the country's medical health college over five years ago and has been stationed in Bimbi ever since. As head of the facility, his duties range to all forms of medical assistance, including maternal health initiatives.

"*Ndili bwino, kaya inu?*" I fumbled with the unpracticed reply, making a mental note to ask Agness how to clarify the pronunciation on our way home.[*]

The chair he sat in creaked as he shifted, bringing his

---

[*] Mzungu is singular the term for a foreigner (azungu is plural), commonly used to describe a Caucasian person. Children particularly love to call out when they spot a mzungu, often chasing our vehicle down the road if they noticed as we passed.

[*] The common greeting translates almost exactly as we say it in Canada. "How are you?", "I'm fine, and you?", "I'm well, thank you", "Good!" I must have practiced this greeting a thousand times throughout my time in Malawi, and I always ended up being laughed at by the people I responded to. I'd look to Agness for help, but she was always laughing with the people too. They appreciated my attempts to greet them but were probably more entertained by the way I butchered the pronunciation.

elbows to rest on the room's central desk. Aaron must have been no older than thirty years old, but he sat before me with weathered experience. His eyes held an endured tiredness, not just from an early morning, but ages of practiced wakefulness and lack of sleep. But they were kind. There was a shine in his eyes that glowed from the depths, reflecting a passionate and fulfilled heart.

Aaron spoke English fluently, and after introducing us, Agness sat on a waiting chair beneath a faded chart and listened to us speak. Clearly eager to share his work, Aaron led the conversation.

"I am the only medical assistant in this facility," he began. "Which means I must see patients day and night—I'm almost always working."

"How many patients do you think you see each day?" I asked, thinking of the overflowing waiting room beyond the hollow door.

He thought for a moment, "About 200, I would say.[*] Most of them are coming in for their drugs or medication, but there are also many who are very sick."

Having collected a high level of training from local universities, medical assistants in Malawi are incredibly valuable. There's a higher population of them, allowing them to reach Malawi in communities where doctors are scarce. Their presence can greatly increase the delivery of health care in these communities. As the only medical assistant in the facility, it was understandable that Aaron's first and heaviest challenge was the workload.

"There is such a lack of resources as well. Sometimes I

---

[*] When I worked as a receptionist for a family doctor in Canada, we would consider it a busy day if the doctor saw around twenty patients. For comparison, Aaron sees almost ten times that amount.

know what must be done to help someone, but I don't have the right tools to do so. In that case, we have to send them to the district hospital, which is much farther away."

I had thought about this before. The hospitals I'm familiar with in Canada are fully equipped to encounter nearly every kind of emergency. In the rare occasions that a patient requires specialized treatment, a bright orange helicopter is ever-ready to transport patients to new hospitals within the hour. Looking around to the four high corners touching brick to tin roof, I wondered how many basic procedures were left untreated here or deferred away simply because of lack of supplies.

This maternal health program only recently provided the means to conduct caesarean sections on delivering mothers, offering elemental training of the procedure to the attending midwives and nurses.

I sat in a moment of shock. In 2015, the global use of caesarean sections had risen to an estimated 27.9 million—nearly doubling the statistics at the start of the century. Of that massive number, central Africa claims only 4.1% of these caesarean births.[iv] While the rest of the world developed and grew in their procedures, villages and communities like Bimbi were being left to their own devices.

How many mothers or infants could have been saved if the resources were as accessible as they should be? How many lives have been lost because this procedure was unable to be performed?

But there was a lack of stitches to heal an open wound. Lack of blood-pressure instruments to determine gestational hypertension or preeclampsia, which are important to be treated on time. Lack of antiseptic to sterilize a small infection. The basic procedures that I expect to be treated with at my own doctor's office are the very things that, when absent here, could be the line between life and death—sickness and health.

"Tell me, Aaron," I asked, knowing he had a story behind his dedication. "Why did you decide to become a medical assistant? It's so much work, but what led you here?"

The chair creaked as he sat back, "I was born into a family where sickness is a part of life. I have a four-year-old daughter as well. I want her to have a healthy life, so I teach her the same things I teach the families in the villages. Brush your teeth every day. Wash your hands. These simple things mean the difference between being healthy and being sick.

"My daughter says that when she grows up, she wants to be like me," Aaron's eyes, which were welcoming to begin with, grew even more gentle. He paused then shook his head, "But I hope she doesn't."

It hurt me to hear those words. Aaron seemed like a loving, dedicated father. A caring man who dedicated nearly every waking hour to the people under his care. But he explained to me that he wouldn't wish his daughter to be under the same pressure that he is, tending to over 200 patients each day. He would rather she take a path in life that keeps her happy and relaxed.

Despite the hours and massive scope of work that Aaron conquers, it's more than clear that he enjoys the challenge.

"I love to see them all," his smile flashed. "It's my passion. To help people and put them back on their feet."

I didn't want to take more time away from Aaron and

the many patients waiting beyond the door, so Agness and I stood and thanked him for his time. He smiled, thanking me instead, insisting that it was his pleasure.

As we emerged from the little office room, another brightly clad mother slipped between the door and the frame, and Aaron was back to work again.

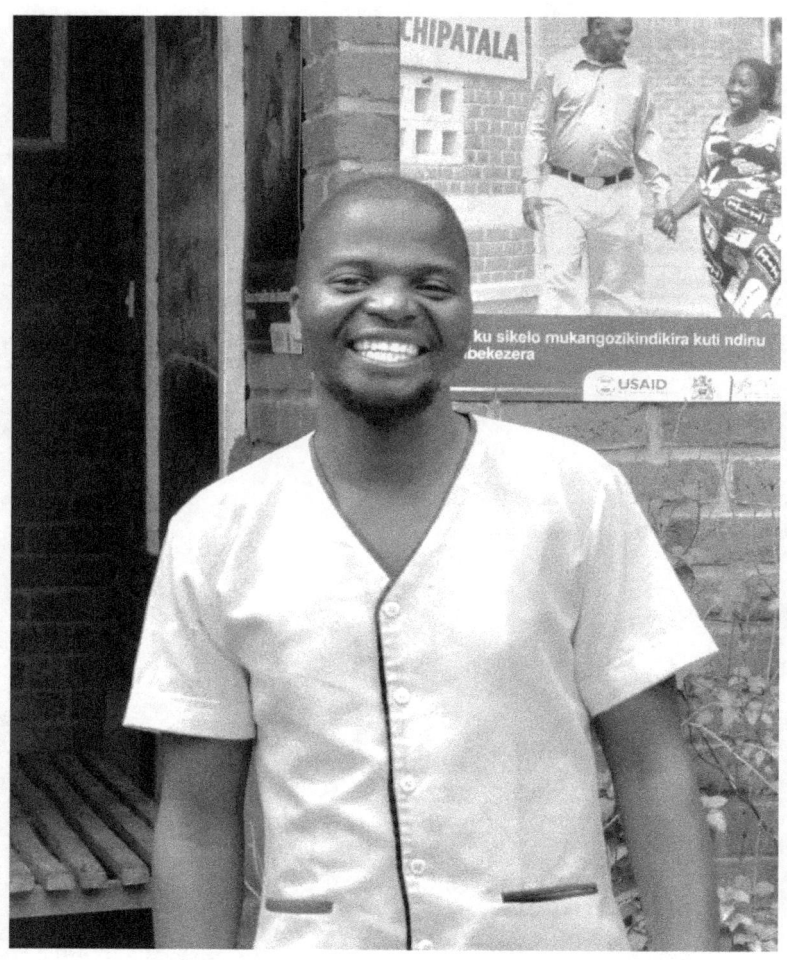

FRANCIS

I met Francis the same day that I spoke with Aaron. He was waiting for me in the second waiting 'room'—this one designated exclusively for the maternity ward. There were about fifteen women waiting here, their colorful *chitenges* decorating the smooth cement benches. A few were carrying little ones strapped tightly to their backs by the same *chitenges* that they had wrapped around their waists.

Francis led me to an open bench, and we sat facing each other.

"I want to thank you for coming," he opened, his deep English consonants rounded by the Chichewa accent. He knew English well enough to let Agness off the hook, so she slipped outside in search of another volunteer she wanted to meet with.

"No, Francis!" I laughed. "It's me who should be thanking you! You've taken the time to speak with me."

He smiled with a humble tilt of his head, "I am happy to help you, sister."

Francis, I decided, was going to be one of my favorite people that I would speak with. He was officially dubbed a nurse at the clinic, but his role encompassed far more than the already complex position carries.

"I am called a nurse, but I really do far more than that. I am also a midwife—I help with deliveries and family planning. I'm an STI treatment provider and I also work with youth-friendly services." He paused, processing his other duties in the clinic. "Oh! I'm also part of the outreach team. I come to the villages and speak to individual households about proper health practices."

I looked around, the clinic was over-populated with patients, confirming the drought of health care providers. How could one man do so much?

"It was not my choice to come here," Francis's head bobbed again, his voice quieting. "But there was such a shortage of nurses. I had to come."

He moved on to tell the extent of what the new maternal health project endeavored to do, and I began to understand his plight. The scope of work was huge. Nurses were receiving further training to deal with various kinds of birthing complications and offer better care for mothers who come for regular checkups throughout their pregnancies. Their funding organization was providing the clinic with delivery kits for women and supplying privacy curtains between beds. They were digging placenta pits so as to safely dispose of the placentas after birth.

There were nutrition plans, garden training, and better breastfeeding practices being taught. Family planning and reproductive education is in development—forefront on the minds of the program participants. The program's purpose is not simply to take the terribly high maternal and infant mortality by the roots, but to completely transform the entire plant.

On top of all his current responsibilities, Francis had

aspirations of his own. "I do not have time for it yet, but I have a great passion to address teenage pregnancy. I want to teach family planning in schools."

Francis was not a shy man, but his posture righted and once modest eyes deepened as he continued to speak. "There are many, many girls who are getting pregnant too young. Even at fifteen years old."

Their pregnancies contributed to the sorrowful cycle in maternal mortality rates. According to UNICEF, 31% of women in Malawi will have given birth to their first child by the time they're eighteen.[v] Concurrently, adolescent pregnancies comprise 25% of all births and 20% of all maternal deaths.[vi]

Not only do these young women step into motherhood before their time, but it forces them to drop out of school. Francis does not yet have any children of his own, but his wife serves as a teacher at a school in a neighboring village. "It is not right that they must drop out of school. I want them to have a future!"

"Francis, why do you suppose so many young people in Malawi seem to be at risk of pregnancies?" Even in the room around us, there were several mothers whose age could not have surpassed eighteen.

"There is a myth that many women believe in Malawi," he began. "That if you study family planning and learn about responsible reproduction, you will never be able to have children—not even in the future."

I couldn't form the words to my next question. My tongue had twisted into shocked silence, a million questions damming my speech. How could a myth like that begin? Were there people who experienced this before, and decided it was true? How were women and men supposed to break the cycle if they couldn't even learn how? How could anyone believe this?

Francis watched my reaction knowingly. He laughed when all I could stammer out was a painful "What?"

He further explained the situation. The belief has no traceable origin, but it is widely spread enough to be causing difficulties when programs attempt to introduce a curriculum into their schools.

Teenage pregnancies in Malawi are particularly dangerous. I spoke with Anke, a German gynecologist and obstetrician a few days later, and asked her about it. Anke and her family had lived in Malawi for some time, where she worked in the district hospital, guiding and teaching the nurses, doctors and midwives in maternal and newborn care practices.

She explained that one of the leading causes in maternal death in teens is that many fifteen-year-old bodies are simply not developed enough to deliver safely. To further this, the hospitals and clinics are not advanced enough to protect them. As of 2015, 1 of every 29 Malawian teenage pregnancies resulted in death. Just ten years prior, that number was 1 in 18.[vii]

Quite often, Anke said, the young mother's cervix has simply not grown enough to make room for a child to pass through. Because many of these women do not have access to caesarian sections, or other adequate care, they will suffer an assortment of complications such as excessive bleeding, uterine rupture, or hemorrhages.

Francis knew all of this. In fact, he had taken part in it first-hand as a midwife technician. As an outreach member, he saw it when he went door to door. As a nurse, he saw it in countless patients. As a Malawian, it surrounds him everywhere as part of the culture.

"One of the challenges is education," he reiterated. "We just need to teach them when they are young."

I will not forget his voice of urgency and empathy. Francis was a man who worked every day to support his patients. He lived away from his wife five days a week in order to keep himself close to the Bimbi Health Facility should any need arise. He took on the title of nurse, the workload of three other positions, and was still driven to do more.

Francis shook my hand with his soft palms and disappeared around the open wall. I stood and walked out in search of Agness, who I found shedding smiles and chatter with a couple more volunteers with the project. There is an endless amount of work to be done, I realized as my conversations took place and I met with more and more Malawians. It could have been so easy for a shadow of doubt to close over the hope that I had. But as I watched Agness with her smart stature and confidence, I realized that sometimes it's far more productive to fuel yourself with the countless stories of successes that have been left in your wake as opposed being stalled by the thousands of icebergs ahead.

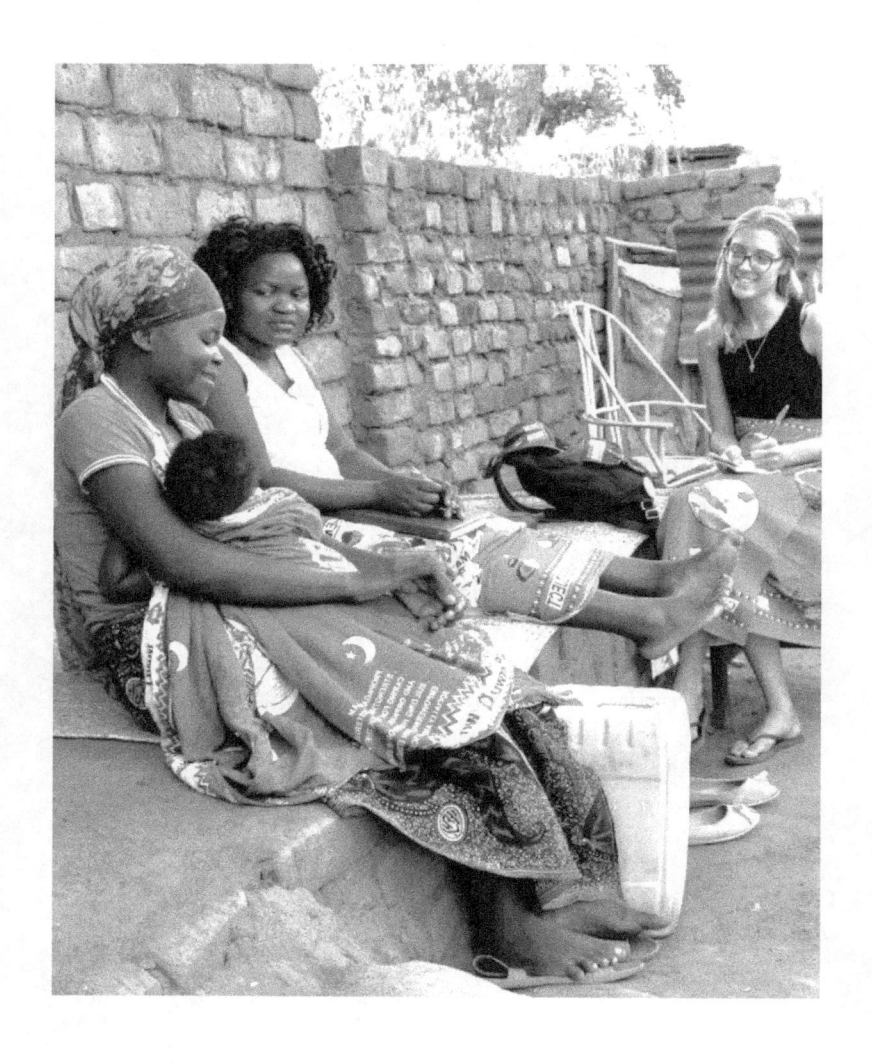

MIRIAM, PARTIMA, BACHALO

Only a few fiery Malawian suns had risen and fallen before I met several ladies living what Francis had just described to me. We didn't conquer the unmarked map of roads and paths until much later in the day, arriving at the village at nearly four in the afternoon. By then, an amber hue had been painted onto every manifest object, varnishing golden glory onto a landscape already so saturated with beauty. We were delayed nearly an hour before setting out because of an unexplained complication with the vehicle's tires.

"Are you *sure* it's on properly?" I joked with our driver after the crew finally managed to replace it. "We might end up walking home from the village if it falls off!"

The team laughed, pestering the driver with more teasing as we hopped into the vehicle. We picked up Agness from her home, apologising for being so late.

She graced us with joyful forgiveness, "I just hope we haven't missed the feeding!"

It turned out that we were not late at all. In fact, it seemed as though the entire village was just congregating as we arrived. A colorful cluster of women danced forward, serenading our approaching team with the most joyful Chichewa verses.

There are so many beautiful noises in this wide world, and one of them is indisputably the unaccompanied harmonization of this group of people—their voices tuned by the open sky and nature's elements, singing with all the joy in their hearts. My generous hosts would offer their porch for a gathering point for a local ladies' Bible study, and I would often place myself near their group just to listen to their elevated Chichewa hymns. On the days I miss the Malawian sun the most, I'll pull out my recordings of their tunes and close my eyes... I don't understand the words, but I understand the song, and my heart is pulled in all directions upwards. What a glorious sound.

The singing group had circled through the few houses nearby, summoning all the families to their congregating place beneath a prodigious tree. Men, children, and women of all ages had come to observe what Agness had called 'the feeding.'

"They are waiting for our team to teach them about feeding their children and making sure they have proper nutrition," Agness leaned towards me. "Every day for twelve days, we will come here and help them use the food groups to make meals for their families."

The program team would weigh all the children in the village before and after the twelve days, keeping track of the immense impact that proper nutrition has—not even two full weeks needs to go by before families can see a difference. Noting such a transformation in a child's weight was more than enough to convince the communities that the program worked.

But Agness whisked me away before I was able to become too interested in their festivities. "There are some ladies I want you to meet."

These women were all young mothers. They were still teenagers when their beautiful little ones were born. And though I spoke to each to them separately, their stories were almost perfect reflections of each other.

I spoke with Miriam first. Her sweet daughter was just under two years old and was cradled in her arms, bold eyes wondering at my presence. Every so often she would become distracted by the squabble of ducks in the courtyard where we sat, but more or less, those wide little eyes were captive and curious about the strange woman speaking a language she couldn't recognize.

Agness introduced us, and Miriam began her story.

"To be honest, I had a very nice pregnancy. After I became pregnant, my partner and I decided we should get married. Since then, I have always had enough food to eat."

Miriam's husband works in the village center at a shop, selling various necessities from the one-room building with an order counter at the front. His absence throughout the day leaves her to do most of the household chores and garden work alone, but she didn't seem to mind.

"It was not until I started labor that I became scared," Miriam said. "I was beginning to lose a lot of blood. My mother and grandmother told me that I should not cry when I went to the hospital—they told me to persevere through the pain."

"Why did they tell you not to cry?" I couldn't imagine being young and scared and in pain with the added pressure to not cry out. But there is a fear among some Malawian women that their doctors will become angry with them if they show their pain. By restraining themselves, they are hoping they receive the best care the doctor can give them.

"I tried to be strong," Miriam touched the cheek of her sweet little one. "But I was still very scared."

She had to stay in the hospital for three days after giving birth. "They were very nice to me. They even gave me extra cloths because of the bleeding."

She had made the comment before, but I had been distracted by imagining her situation. I couldn't begin to put myself in her place—terrified for her own life, terrified for her child's life, and in the most amount of pain she's ever been in. Yet through it all, forbidden to make any sound of anguish for fear she might diminish her chances of optimal care.

But I heard her comment this time: 'They even gave me cloths because of the bleeding.' It rang in my ears and echoed through my mind. There are so many moments in my life, in my travels and all the strangers that I befriend where I am reminded of the depth of cultures so different than my own.

I couldn't imagine being in a position where being treated in a hospital was surprising, or even notable, for that matter. I can appreciate it, but I cannot imagine it. But what broke my heart was how she placed so much emphasis on her receiving extra cloths. Of course, it was not that she valued them that broke my heart, but that Malawi was in a place of such disparity where such kindness was so remarkable. I couldn't voice my fear—did she think that such 'generosity' was because she persevered through the pain?

Partima, another young mother I met, faced a similar

struggle. Being so young and so new to motherhood, she wasn't sure what to expect.

"She was in labor for almost two days before she made it to the hospital," Agness explained to me that Partima, like Miriam, had a very difficult birth. "She was too small for the baby to come on its own."

After hours of bleeding, pain, and excruciating labor, Partima was finally transferred from the Bimbi clinic to the district hospital. "When I arrived, the doctors informed me that they would have to cut part of my cervix so that there would be room to deliver her," I looked to Partima and the little one pulled close to her breast and wondered what kind of thoughts would have been running through her mind. But this young face was so seasoned by reality that it seemed less concerned than I did. She cared for her daughter, just over a year old, with the truest and realest love.

It was Bachalo, a twenty-year-old mother of a two-year-old curiosity, who offered the blunt explanation that was echoed by both Miriam and Partima.

"It was a mistake to have a child so young," Her complete adoration for her little one was unquestionable, but Bachalo was able to acknowledge that she wasn't prepared for motherhood. "It was too painful, and I was simply not ready."

All three of the young women had to drop out of school to facilitate raising a child and caring for a new family. Each of them took their difficult experiences as an opportunity to advocate the implications of having unprotected sex. I asked Bachalo if she had ever received any lessons in family planning, or sex education while she was still in school.

"I did, but I didn't listen to it. Now I'm telling all of my friends to wait. I tell them, 'Don't get into a relationship unless you're ready!'"

Contraceptives are not always available for many men and women in the villages, so the ladies advocate for abstinence until the time is right. Agness explained to me that it's a painful process to try to convince men and women to use contraceptives even if they are available.

"It's one of two reasons," Agness tapped the tips of her fingers, counting the ways. "They don't truly understand the consequences of unprotected sex, and they don't want to alter the sensation of it by using external contraceptives like condoms."

The birth control pill is an uncommon prescription, particularly for women who live deeper in the Malawian landscape.

"I think I may want another child at one time," Miriam's young voice was clear and unfiltered. "But not for a long time. For now, I'm too afraid to have another one."

These young women had nothing but love for their garbling children, even with the knowledge that their own futures are now so limited. Miriam, Partima, and Bachalo are fortunate to have their own lives and their babies' health, and are hopeful, despite their disadvantaged circumstances. An early exit from school results in narrowed opportunities, particularly for women in Malawi.

Agness cooed and chattered to the little ones, wrapped in their mother's support. In the yard, I watched ducks splashing in a metal bowl, bean sprouts dusting the garden green, young eyes poking through the gaps in the fence;

these sights too quickly blind the ladies with familiarity, but I drank it in with appreciation.

"But it's exciting—each morning is new. I'm learning so much every single day." Bachalo scooped up her child in a torn yellow dress and held her tenderly. So much was lost, yet so much is gained.

Eventually our conversations ended, and the ladies joined the festivities back in the village. I saw them chatting with their friends as they watched the nutrition program continue, their heads tossed back and shoulders bouncing as they laughed at the presenter's antics.

Little children ran about, some positioned at the very front of the group, watching with wonder as the program turned into entertainment and educational skits. I watched from afar, sitting next to Agness as she laughed along. Bachalo, Partima, and Miriam were just three young mothers out of an entire village out of an entire country. Their lives were so drastically changed at such a young age, yet they pressed forward with full hope and joy.

The sun was nearly set by the time we gathered ourselves to leave. As I was walking back to the truck, I turned one last time back to the trees where the crowd was dispersing.

I caught Miriam's eyes and they shined at me.

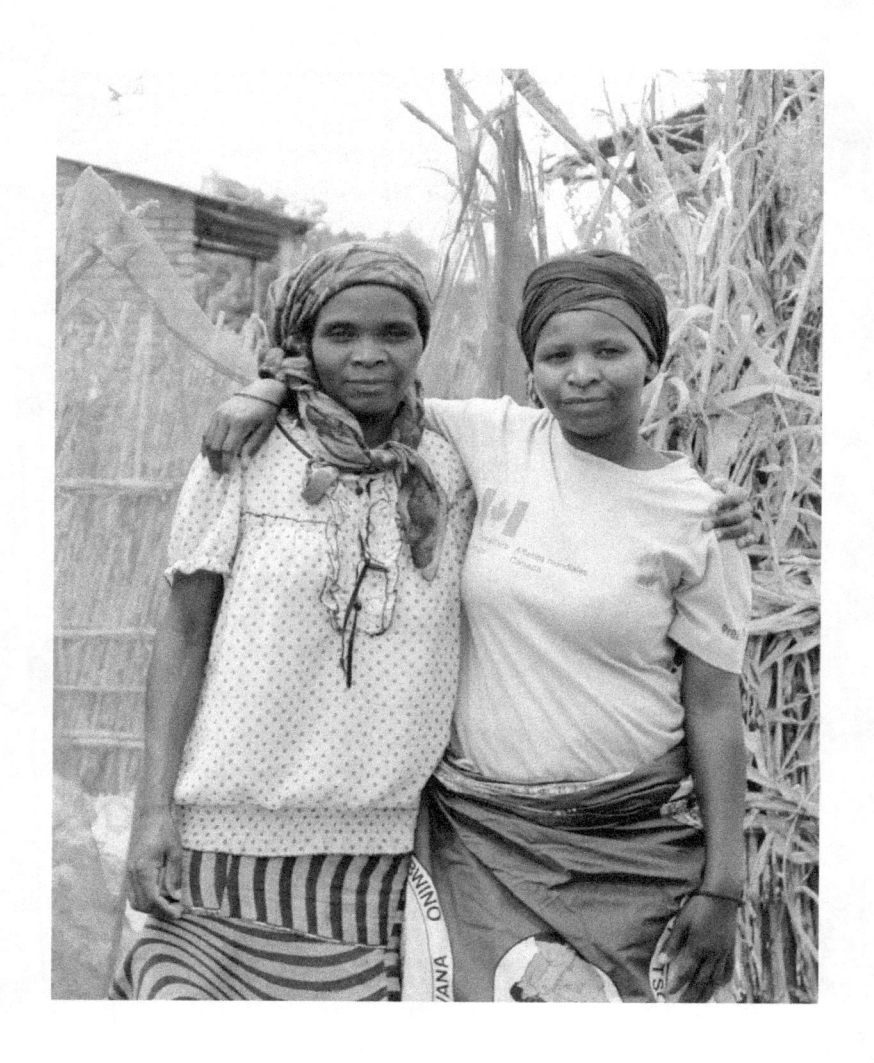

GLADYS

"This is Kathleen."

"Here is Catrina, from Canada."

"Please meet Cattie, she has a few questions for you!"

Agness introduced me with a different name nearly every time we met someone new. The sequence of consonants and vowels that my English name is comprised of are evidently very difficult for the Chichewa tongue to pronounce.[*] I had considered deriving a nickname for myself so poor Agness wouldn't struggle so much, but I was beginning to enjoy discovering how many ways my name could be interpreted. She would interrupt herself now and again— "Your name is so difficult to say!"—and I would laugh, grateful that she even tried.

Today I was Katya of Canada, meeting with Gladys of Malawi. Her village was one that fell under the jurisdiction of the Bimbi Health Facility, and subsequently the care of the PROMISE maternal health program. Gladys was a mother of nine, her children ranging between nineteen

---

[*] I had not yet figured this out on my first expedition to Malawi, and consequently spent a fair amount of time trying to help the drivers, translators, and other people that I met learn to correctly pronounce my name. Eventually they would say a name so assuredly that I would collapse and let them have it. By the end of my stay, I'm pretty sure nobody knew who I was anymore.

and three years of age. Though I didn't understand the words she spoke until Agness translated them for me, I could hear her quiet assuredness and experience beyond her years in the softness of her voice.

"I was born here, and I will grow old here," she gestured to the dry village, a scattering of houses and trees. A goat bleated and tip-tapped past our trio, its frayed rope dragging along the ground beside it.

Gladys has been a mother for nearly twenty years, but it's only been the past three that she has learned more than she has ever known in terms of providing and helping her children grow. One of the greater contributing factors to the high statistics in maternal mortality and child mortality is the lack of awareness surrounding proper nutrition practices. In fact, according to a 2011 study, over 36% of Malawian households lacked access to sufficient food sources, resulting in an estimated 47% of children to be stunted in their growth.[viii]

I saw previously that Malawian diets are not enough to be considered full—lacking in both quality and quantity. It's something that nearly all charitable organizations in the country strive, in one way or another, to address. And because it's such a large contributor to general health, it's particularly important for mothers, fathers, and families to know proper nutrition practices if not to promote their own health, but also maternal and child health. It's a massive component to the maternal health project that I was following, and Gladys was more than happy to show off her newfound knowledge.

Agness taught me on several occasions that the massive disparity of proper nutrition practices among families did not stem from a neglectful nature of the men and women in Malawi but rather a genuine ignorance of best practices. Gladys and many like her are keen to learn and implement better strategies when it comes to the health of their children. In the past two years, Gladys has taken and run with nearly all of the strategies the program has taught her.

"You must come see my garden," She invited me through the torn mosquito-net gate and into the corn-stalk enclosure. "We learned about the importance of the six food groups.[*] They taught us how to keep a garden so that we will always have access to fruits and vegetables. I used to pay 150 Kwacha each day on veggies for my children, but now it all comes from here!"[*]

The garden was a calculated mosaic of fresh growth. Little sprouts and green leaves were poking through the dry clay in careful rows and sections. Agness took me around the plot, identifying each of the plants.

"These are pumpkins." She squatted to inspect the large leaves just inches off the ground. "And these are her green beans. Do you see the tomato plants growing here? And notice the sweet potatoes too—have you ever had okra before?"

I saw Agness's joy in the growth of the garden, Gladys's pride in her hard work, and the other villagers who had gathered to support. They all took part in explaining the particular vegetables they were able to

---

[*] Countries will designate their recommended food groups according to the specific needs in their population. The Malawian Ministry of Health outlines six: Staples, Fats, Animals, Legumes, Vegetables, and Fruits.

[*] One hundred fifty Malawian Kwacha is equivalent to thirty cents. It may seem insignificant to you or me, but when your net income is around $500/year (or less), every penny counts.

grow in Malawi's climate, the importance that these gardens had among the communities, and the significant impact that they had on overall nutrition with an excitement brought on from the complete assuredness of the success of the program.

Having a garden in their own backyard means that families can become self-sufficient; growing their own produce saves money, but also acts as a way to ensure that quality, nutritious food is readily available to them.

"It saves them trips to the marketplace too—the accessibility of food is greater for them than any other way," Agness smiled.

Gladys continued her Chichewa narrative, pointing to more plants and gently touching their growing leaves, a proud grin lighting up her wizened face. She showed me her goat droppings, used as fertilizer, and the sturdy corn fence she used to keep those very goats out.

"Before, my children were malnourished and very weak. But I've learned ways to make sure that my children are properly fed and strong. Now they are able to stay in school!"

I asked Gladys about her older children and if she was able to communicate what she was learning to them, but her voice quieted in response. "My older children have moved far away. I can't teach them what I'm learning now." But she can and does teach the children still in her household, and she teaches the rest of her village as well.

Later, as Agness and I watched the cloud of red dust swirl behind the retreating vehicle, I tried to think about the position Gladys was in. Her first several children were already married with children of their own, quite possibly the same age as her youngest children.

Would her grandchildren be receiving the same care that Gladys now knows is necessary to give? Do her older, married children have the same opportunities and knowledge that their mother has? Gladys bore and raised all nine of her children in the same village, and though she still raises the younger ones, how can she pass that care forward to her older ones?

My own mother and I are very close, and though I live a considerable distance from home, Mom still acts as my number one confidant. She is my advice-giver and story-sharer. We discuss life and struggles and joys and knowledge. We go to each other for guidance and seek each other out for updates. I know Mom will call me when she needs to tell me her ideas, her advice, and what new inspirations she adopts. But our mediums of communication are endless.

Gladys has infinitely more limitations than my own mother and I do. From distance to infrastructure and culture itself—I could see the sadness in Gladys as she described her inability to share her knowledge—her life-giving knowledge—to her own children.

Yet this mama presses on. She imparts her new nutritional and hygienic practices to the children that are still under her care. She teaches them the six food groups and shows them just how important their backyard gardens really are. And it's working. Her little ones are stronger than ever, as are the rest of the children in the village!

"We haven't had a cholera outbreak, or any disease like it, come through the village in over two years," Gladys explained, flashing her peaceful smile to a friend who stopped to listen. Their lives are changing. Slowly and surely, their hope is growing.

"What do I hope for my children?" Gladys repeated my question, barely pausing before she answered. "I want them to be healthy. And I want them to be wise."

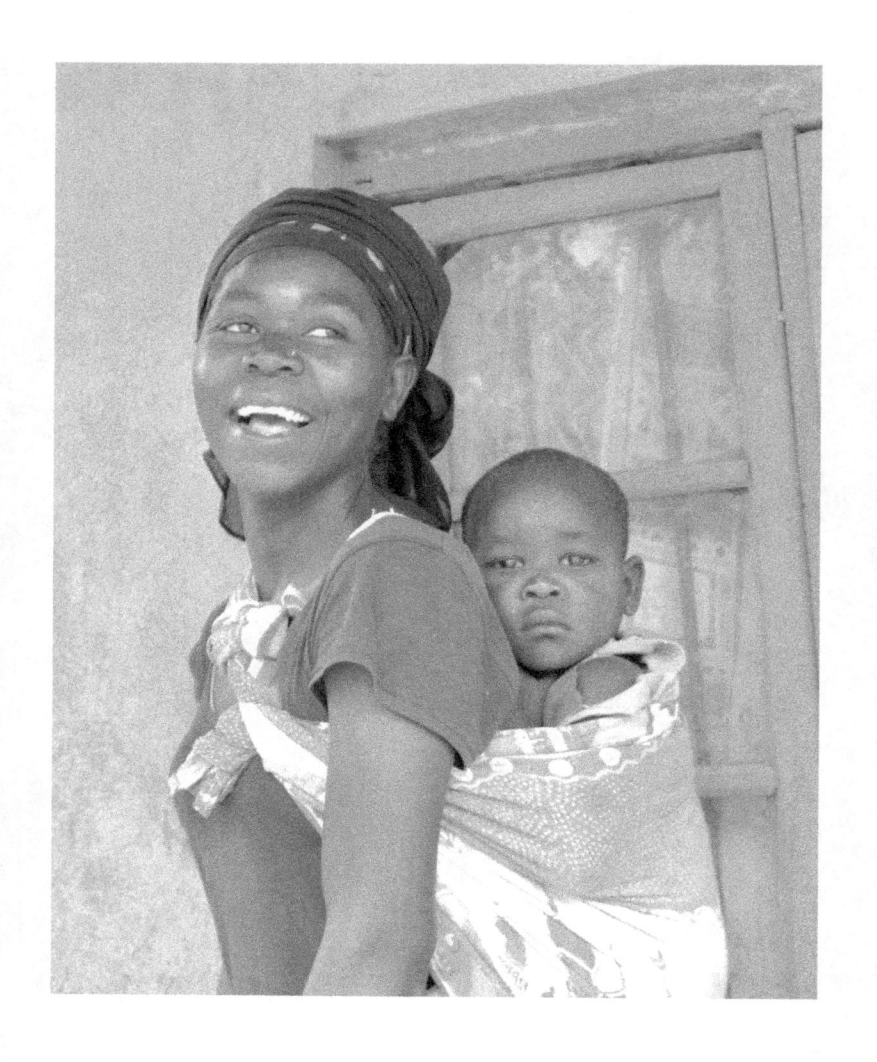

KILATU

It rained that evening. The first rain the Malawian soil has touched in nearly five months. I could hear the thunder rolling over the rocks and dry ground of the Zomba plateau for hours before the clouds finally released their grip on the massive drops of life. I could smell the rain before I heard it singing on the tin roof. The lightning scared the breeze through the open windows, and it brought along the comforting scent of damp dust and breathing trees.

It was far too early for the rainy season to begin: the tears of the sky barely penetrated the sun-baked ground before it was all over. But it was enough to offer a moment of relief from the roasting Malawian air. It was a promise of the approaching season. The sky was saying to us, "Just you wait, there's more of this to come! I'll bring the rains soon." The grass was painted green once again—if only for a moment.

But as I lay in bed listening to the sporadic melody of the tiny drummers on the tin roof, I thought about Kilatu and her three little children. I wondered if she also saw the parallels between the nourishing rain and the nourishment that her children now experience—an infusion of hope and a promise of what is to come.

Kilatu is the mother of three boys, with a straw-swept yard and clay-smeared walls. Her windows have ocean-blue shutters and white chipped paint. Agness was the one who pointed out the clay-smeared walls smiling, "It makes me so happy—see they've done it on all the houses!"

It was true, nearly all of the red brick and clay buildings had a foot of fresh gray clay spread evenly around the base of it. The village looked clean, smart and sanitary. "That was what I advised them to do last time I was here. I'm so glad they did!"

The smearing of clay is multifunctional. Its primary purpose is to fill in faults and cracks in the burnt-brick walls protecting the building from cracking and falling apart.[ix] Agness explained that it also serves as a sanitation method— sealing the ground and base of the house from more particles entering, allowing the area to be easily swept and kept clean.

I loved watching Agness proudly admire the homes, peeking through doors here and there to see the inside. Her cheeks carried an unrelenting smile, spreading like wildfire to the rest of us.

Kilatu was absolutely beautiful. Her eyes carried humble grace and a glint of adventure. When she began her soft story, I started to understand hope in a whole new light.

"My first child was very malnourished and unhealthy. He only weighed twelve kilograms when he was five years old. He was a very ill child, even after they treated him for malnutrition. He would be losing weight instead of gaining it," Kilatu began, waiting for Agness to finish translating her words to me.

I did quick math in my head. The average, healthy weight for a five-year-old child is about 18.4 kilograms,[x] which meant that Kilatu's firstborn was missing nearly a third of the weight that he should have had.[*] Her son would be among the 1.07 million children under five years in Malawi who suffer from chronic malnutrition,[xi] making a narrow escape from being among many little ones who are lost because of it. Such malnourishment makes them susceptible to disease, illness, and bacteria. Their weakened bodies and damaged immune systems can be taken out by the smallest bug. At that point in his life, the simple equation was obvious: Kilatu's son was in danger.

"I wasn't content with the malnourishment program we tried for him. We were seeing no change—my son was still losing weight!" Kilatu paused as the wind swept a sudden dust devil through our conversation. We dove for cover, shielding our faces from the golden red dirt and other debris carried towards the sky.

It only lasted a moment, but true to her nature, Agness had been laughing the whole time. The wind must have brought a new energy too, because the two women erupted in Chichewa banter, teasing each other about the dust. I grinned, watching the mini twister break against a neighboring house and shaking its carnage off of my *chitenge*.

Agness leaned towards me, "Those are common this time of year," she broke off with laughter, brushing a little stick off her shoulder. "Oh, there's dust everywhere!"

It was Kilatu that brought us back to the conversation, anxious to conclude her story and display the improvements to her children and their health. "I have learned so much about nutrition now. This new program has taught us so

---

[*] For those of you who are terrible Canadians like me who don't understand kilograms as a unit of measurement, Kilatu's firstborn *should* have weighed about 40.5 lbs in order to align to a healthy weight for his age. Instead, he weighed 26 lbs.

much. They taught me about exclusive breastfeeding, which I had never heard of before."

Agness had explained to me what exclusive breastfeeding meant prior to meeting Kilatu, but my mind still spun, tossing around questions like the dust storm that just passed through.

Exclusive breastfeeding is a practice that is advertised throughout many maternal health programs in countries like Malawi. Its importance is stressed upon the mothers like Kilatu and her community upon the discovery that may mothers were simply unaware of how harmful their current breastfeeding practices were. Simply put, exclusive breastfeeding is as the name suggests: to feed a child frequently, and to only feed breast milk, until their children are at least six months of age.

Malawi's current rate of exclusive breastfeeding is at a mere 61%, which rapidly decreases as the child grows. By the time a child is four months old, that figure nearly halves.[xii]

"I didn't know that I should be breastfeeding my child for so long. Before, I would start to give them food at maybe three months. But I know now that isn't right," Kilatu also shared with me that she was equally unaware of the importance of frequent feedings. "I didn't know they needed to be fed so often!"

It's similar in a lot of women like Kilatu. There's an unawareness that their growing little ones would require multiple feedings throughout the day—across the country many women will often go an entire day without breastfeeding their children. Agness had to explain me out of the shock I was in when I discovered it.

"That's part of the culture," Agness said. "Often a mother

won't make the connection that even though they do not need to eat so frequently, their child does. If a mother skips breakfast, their child is likely not to be fed then either. We've had to teach them that their growing child needs to be fed many times throughout the day—and it works! Now they make sure they are breastfeeding their children for longer and for multiple times each day."

The results are life-changing in the most literal interpretation.

"My second child was the same way as my first. But I know so much more about nutrition now. I learned to frequently breastfeed, and to only breastfeed until they reach a certain age. And I have learned about the food groups. Peanuts are a substitute for protein. This little one here is much healthier than the first two were. You can tell because of his appearance." It was true—her little boy strapped to her back was a healthy kind of plump. He stared around at Agness and I as we spoke with his mother, not understanding but happily resting against his mother regardless.

Kilatu is by no means a neglectful mother. I considered her circumstances as I lay under the mosquito net listening to the tin-song lullaby of the rain that evening. Her children were not so malnourished because she refused to feed them or because she couldn't handle the responsibility of their care. Can you blame someone who just doesn't know? Can you hold them accountable to their culture of miseducation and inexperience?

Kilatu's children are now healthier than they've ever been. Her youngest son was born into her newfound knowledge and will hopefully never feel the effects of malnutrition. The gladdened mother has discovered the joys of sustainable nutrition, of keeping her backyard garden, and of exclusive breastfeeding.

And though there are so many little ones who aren't as fortunate, I was thankful for the bright and gentle eyes of Kilatu, and the hope that she emanated from her demeanor, encouraging me to my core.

The orchestra of water stopped playing outside, and I fell asleep listening to the hungry soil drinking in the nourishment of the first rainfall.

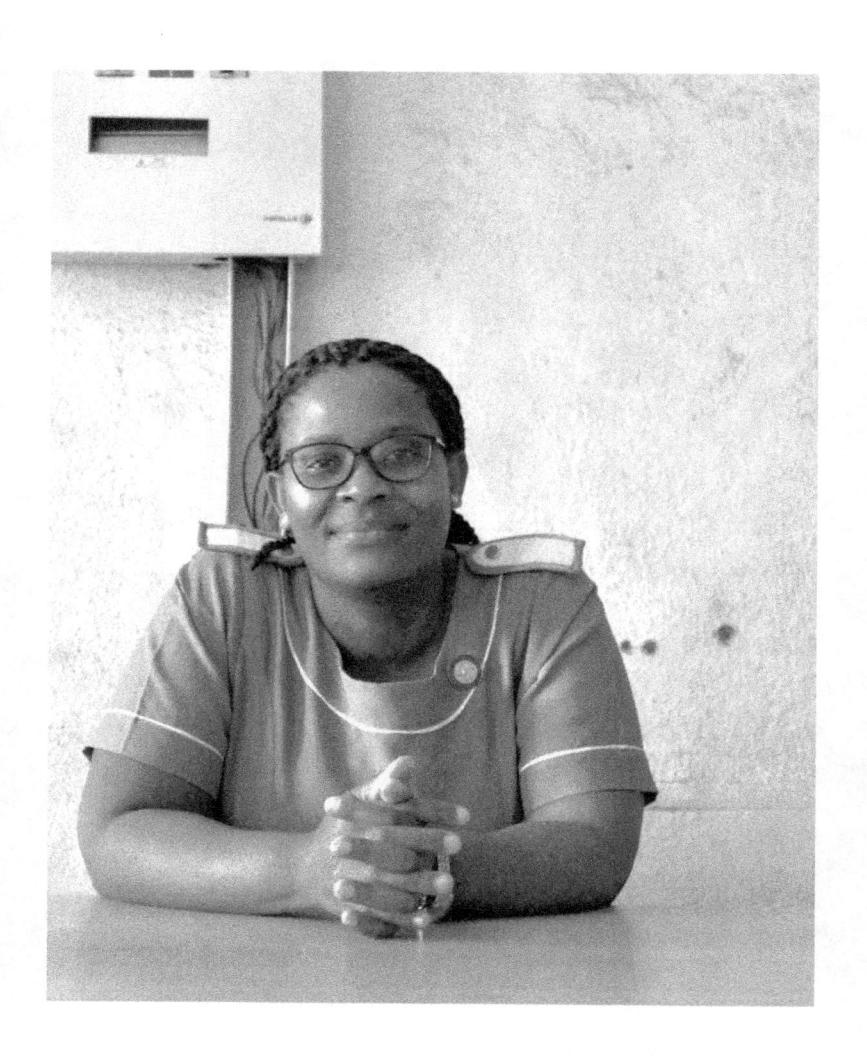

MRS. MVULA

Mrs. Mvula is the exact type of woman I would imagine filling her role. From the conducting stature of her shoulders to the articulate direction with which she spoke, I doubt there is anyone better suited for her position.

We met in the Headquarters of Health in Zomba, offices attached to the Zomba District Hospital. Agness had taken me there to speak with the District Health Officer (DHO) so we could inform him of our mission with this book and courteously ask for his permission and advice. He wasn't around when we arrived, but we spoke with his representatives and they gave us their full support.

The offices were like most of the other buildings in Malawi—cement walls and floors, with a large tin roof. Instead of glass, the windows were filled with an open brick design, blocking most of the hot sun's rays, but allowing for air flow and wind to pass through. As we exited the DHO's office, Agness and I stumbled into a man she knew well.

"*Muli bwanji!*" he said, his bright eyes teasing me. He waited to see if I had practiced my greeting.

"*Muli bwanji! Kaya inu?*" But it seemed that no matter how much I practiced the pronunciation, they always laughed.

We finished the greeting, and he disappeared around the corner, trailing the end of the last chuckling vowel, "*Zikomo-*

o-o." [*]

I turned to Agness, shaking my head with exaggerated exasperation, "I'll never get it!"

She grinned, leading me through the door into next office. One lonely desk in the middle of the room shared the space with countless boxes and other assorted items being stored. Mrs. Mvula spoke perfect English, so Agness's translating expertise wasn't necessary. She introduced us and slipped out of the room to meet with another worker.

Mrs. Mvula was eloquent and poised. She was the kind of woman who knew what she was talking about, inspiring confidence in every syllable she spoke. "It is not always easy to train midwives. Imparting knowledge is simple, but to impart skill, that is difficult," she began, introducing the complex nature of what she does.

As a Midwife Specialist and Master Trainer, Mrs. Mvula not only delivers infants and trains other midwives, but she is one of few Master Trainers in Malawi who have the wholesome task to instruct midwives how to teach other midwives. A teacher's teacher, if you will.

With her own education in Integrated Maternal and Newborn Health, Mrs. Mvula is currently equipping over forty-five clinicians with the skills they need to address serious complication and medical conditions in pregnancy and delivery. Though she's been a midwife for over twenty years, she explained that it's never easy to teach someone

---

[*] *Zikomo* = Thank You. It also is used for 'hello,' 'goodbye,' 'okay,' and basically any other filler. If there's one word that is essential to know in Malawi, it's this one. If Canadians are known to say 'sorry,' then '*zikomo*' would be the Chichewa equivalent.

to be skilled in her profession; learning facts and concepts of birth and delivery are one thing, but cultivating talent and aptitude for the pressures of midwifery are another.

Malawi suffers a painful lack of experts, with over 17% of deliveries still unattended by skilled birth attendants, whether it be a midwife, nurse, or otherwise. [xiii]

Training women and men in the ways of delivering a child is incredibly valuable for the preservation of life throughout the country, Mrs. Mvula taught me. The more trained clinicians that can make their way into all the villages, the more fearful and tearful lives can be saved.

Trainings consist of anything from basic delivery to breach birth and caesarian sections.

At the same time, Mrs. Mvula is working hard to encourage her patients and trainees with the importance of regular checkups. "We need to be equipping women with knowledge." She brought her expert hands to her face. "Mothers would be coming to us in the late second or third trimesters with no previous appointments!"

How can the health of a mother and her child be monitored and preserved if there have been no previous checkups? By that time, any complications that could have been dealt with earlier have already irreversibly manifest themselves.

I learned that the Bimbi Health Facility and so many others like it are offering 'birthing kits' to any mother who came within her first trimester. It was a small incentive for the mothers to come, but it was effective. Birthing kits are essentially all the items that mothers are required to provide when they deliver in the clinics. The kits are equipped with an assortment of items including plastic sheeting, soap, disposable gloves, cord clamps and razors.

Also within the kits are reusable sanitary napkins and diapers, face cloths, and a washing basin.

I was shocked when I learned that women are meant to provide nearly all of these items on their own when they were giving birth, and how those simple items can make all the difference between a safe and unsafe delivery. Sometimes the simplest birthing kit can save both the lives of mother and child.

Mrs. Mvula isn't just an expert; she carries a contagious passion for her craft as well. "I initially was trained as a nurse, but I fell in love with midwifery. I want to contribute to the health of this country—to the health of women and children."

With two beautiful little ones of her own, Mrs. Mvula's compassion for the mothers, and her joy in her profession is unquestionable. "I even dream about delivery," She laughed. "You could call me in the middle of the night, and I could tell you exactly what you need to do."

Mrs. Mvula couldn't stick around and speak with me for very long—she was scheduled for another training just after my interruption of her day.

"*Zikomo*, Mrs. Mvula," I said, teasing her with a smile. She laughed and waved me off, sending me out of her shared office and back out on the dusty road.

I'm eternally thankful for the passion of people like her that remind me of the hope for the women and children of Malawi. Mrs. Mvula's motherly disposition would bring a confidence to any families that were under her care. She had a stature of assurance, humbly and securely bearing the image of a champion of midwifery. In a place where maternal health is a major issue overlooked too long, I was thankful that Malawi had a woman like Mrs. Mvula to fight for their lives and fight for their health.

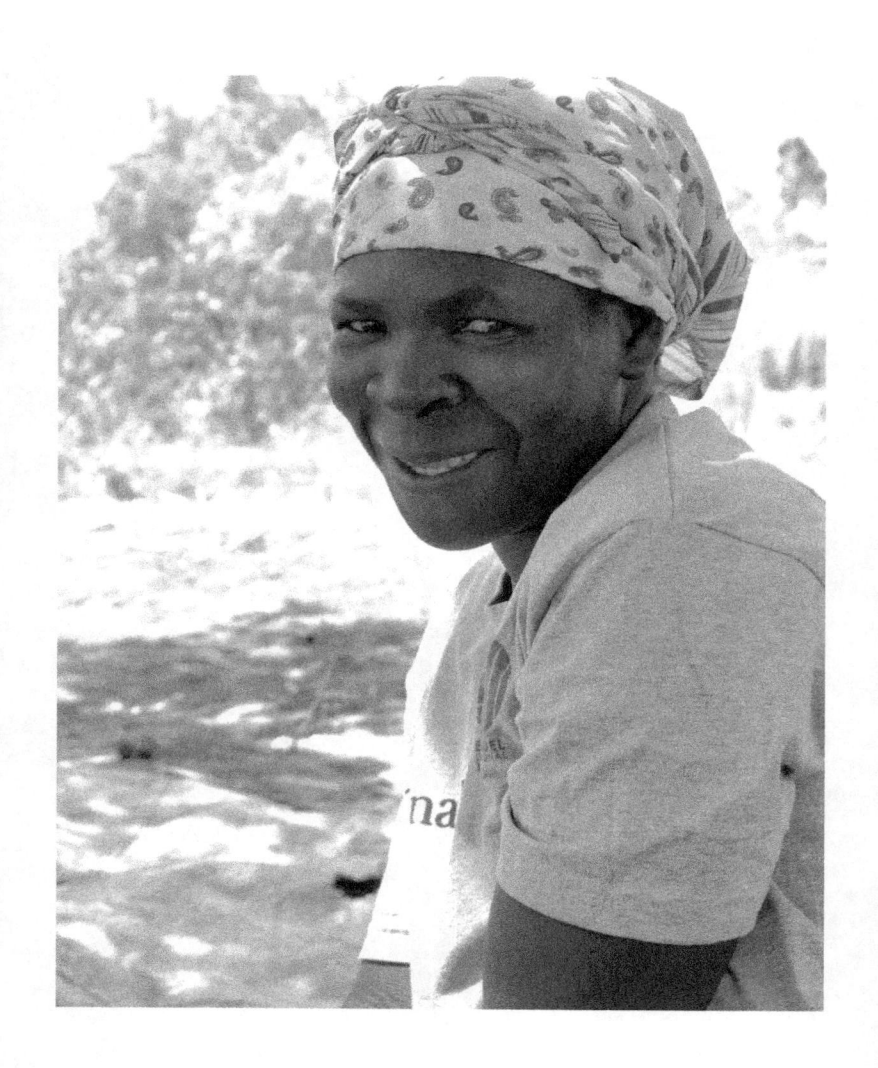

FYNES

When I was a child, I used to spend every second of my time outdoors.[*] In the summertime, our mom would practically expel us from the house until it was time to come back in for lunch or dinner. So long as the weather held up, my brothers and I would happily spend hours coming up with all sorts of ways to entertain ourselves. I knew every inch of the woods behind our house. The two-story tree fort my dad built for us was our constant fortress. I was forever dragging myself home from frog hunts and bike falls.

But I have a particularly vivid memory of the dust at the bottom of our driveway. The road we lived on was crudely paved, and there would always be piles of sand and fine dust pooling at the edges, where the grass met the asphalt. I would often sit in the dust watching my brothers play ball hockey or doing tricks on their bikes and make piles of the sand at the bottom of the driveway.

I'd scoop it up and sift out the larger pebbles, letting the cloud of chalk float away. I'd smooth it out and write

---

[*] Let's face it. As an adult, I *still* attempt to spend every second of my time outdoors. Every free moment I get is spent in precious retreat outdoors. I'm alive when the sunshine's on my face and the fresh air is on my skin.

my name, soft indentations of undecipherable letters in the dirt. I'd make anthills and roadways and kingdoms out of imagination and dust. My bare skin and shoeless feet would come inside at the end of the day, shades of chalky dust lighter than they already were.

With no other explanation than that of a child's mind, I absolutely loved playing in the dust at the side of the road.

I met a mama who gave birth there.

At 4 a.m. on the side of the dust-filled Malawian road, sobbing in pain and gasping in fear. She gave birth to a tiny baby girl. It was there, on the same morning on the same side of the road in the same gasps of pain that the precious little one died.

The mama's name was Fynes, already a mother of three. She lived in a small village about an hour walk from the Bimbi Health Facility. On a bicycle, Fynes could be there in just under half an hour; a vehicle would take only seven minutes. In a Canadian sense of geography, she actually lived rather close to the facility. But for a woman in labor, with no mode of transportation—and at 4 a.m.—the facility was an exact lifetime away.

"We delayed going to the hospital because there was no transportation. We were waiting for the neighbor's oxcart to arrive, but it was taking too long," Fynes was playing with a mango as she spoke, but her voice was strong and unwavering. I watched Agness's face as Fynes told her story, the creases filled with compassion, understanding, and empowerment. Agness loved her task of translating just as much as I loved her for it; the stories we encountered were fueling mission and purpose and hope within Agness, and I felt privileged to see it.

Many of our conversations with the people in Malawi would often take place with an audience. The community loved to be part of our conversations, listening and observing our questions and responses. There were always children watching, and other mamas to offer their support. But knowing what stories we were encountering that day, Agness wisely segregated ourselves. We spoke privately with Fynes on a pleated mat in the shade of a mango tree, separate from the general audience. I was grateful, because it allowed for the privacy of sharing such an emotional and difficult story.

Fynes continued her story, "My mother-in-law and brother helped me into the cart once the team finally arrived." She was accompanied by a few other friends who were also awake to support her.

The Malawian sunrise is typically consistent throughout the year, the golden crest peeking over the horizon between 5 and 6 a.m. in accordance with the season. Fynes's 4 a.m. journey towards the hospital would have been done in the navy-blue darkness of night, the promised sun extinguishing the deep black and softening the hues ever so slightly. But that night will forever be dark for Fynes.

"There were so many delays. We were delayed leaving for the hospital. We were delayed on arriving. I was not far from the facility when I did finally give birth." But understandably, Fynes was not accompanied by any skilled birth attendants on the side of the road. Her family, though caring, were completely unaware of how to deliver a child.

"Then there were more delays. They delayed cutting the umbilical cord; they weren't sure how to do it. They also didn't know that I still had to deliver the placenta, so that was delayed too." Fynes glanced at me, and I suddenly was very aware of what her perception of me would be.

Who was I, a *mzungu*, to show up in the middle of nowhere with a pen and camera and ask about the death of a beloved child? My questions were clearly derived from a privileged understanding of health and maternal care, and despite my research and intentional awareness, it was unavoidable that I had no experience in the matter. For the hundredth time that day, I was thankful for Agness and the filter she provided my questions.

Fynes continued to share her story with me, however, and I made as much as an effort I could to make evident the compassion and heartbreak I had for her despite our language barrier.

"At some point, I became unconscious. I stopped feeling anything and was unaware of everything going on around me." At some point between the birth of her daughter and the full rise of the sun, Fynes was taken from the Bimbi Health Facility to Zomba District Hospital. The placenta was eventually removed, but the little one had already passed away.

Fynes had to stay an additional three weeks at Zomba's hospital, undergoing various treatments to save her own life after the infection and loss of blood caused by the retained placenta. Sicker than she had ever been, Fynes confessed that the experience left her traumatized and fearful.

"I never expected this to happen. Nobody ever does. That experience really changed me," she faltered. "I was so scared to have another child. I waited for five years after that experience."

Today, Fynes is the happy mother of five children, proud and excited for their lives. "I take good care of them. I make sure they're healthy and are eating the right kinds of food." It was powerful to hear her heartbreaking story, the slow and steady recounting of her most painful experience. It was equally powerful to see the woman she is now—the smiling and laughing mama, soaring with pride and wisdom.

Later, Agness and I were waiting for our driver to come and retrieve us from the shade of the mango tree, and the audience we had sent away returned. Agness chatted in her ever-friendly way with the women in the village, and I listened, absent-mindedly tracing my name into the red dirt of the ground. For a moment, I was seven years old again, watching my brothers pass the orange ball-hockey puck back and forth.

I snapped back to the present again, the roadside dirt with a whole new meaning, and I wondered just how many other women had also delivered in the dust.

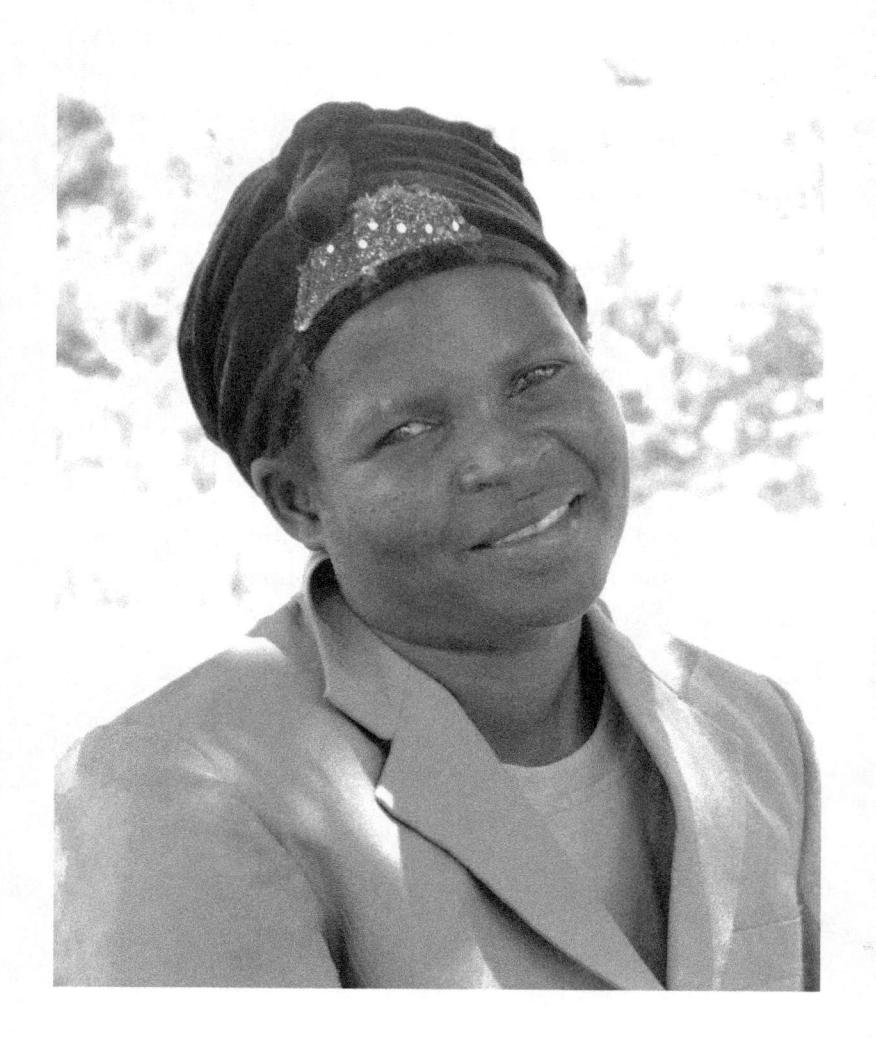

MARIA

Admittedly, I was nervous for this day. I had told Agness at the very beginning that I wanted to speak to these mamas, but I hadn't fully readied myself for their stories. How does one prepare to talk with mothers who have lost their children?

I knew that their stories were valuable—critical to the overall message of this book. But I was nervous to ask the questions I needed to ask. How does one gently, gracefully, and compassionately ask a complete stranger to tell me how her baby died? How do you graciously prod for the details? I was humbled yet again, impressed, and slightly taken aback by their openness. They offered the details before I even asked. I was afraid to come off as insensitive, yet these mamas seemed to be more or less at peace with their stories.

The harsh reality of death is not foreign to mothers and children in Malawi. With a recorded neonatal mortality rate[*] of 20 deaths for every 1,000 live births and

---

[*] Neonatal Mortality Rates are a calculation of how many children pass away within the first 28 days since their birth. Infant Mortality Rates are calculated up to 1 year since birth. These numbers have been on a steady decline since data tracking began; in 1965 the Infant Mortality Rate in Malawi was at a staggering 211 of every 1,000 children.

31 of every 1,000 children dying before their first birthday, these tragedies are not surprising to the communities, though never less heartbreaking.[xiv]

Maria brought Agness and I mangos when she came to speak with us. They were washed in a tin bowl, a tough green skin hiding the sour fruit. I had been advised by several people that it would be for the best to withhold eating foods in the villages for fear of contamination, bugs, or even bacteria that my body isn't used to.

But I have a character that when it comes to sweet food offered to me, I can never say no. When Agness passed the bowl my way, I didn't even consider rejecting the fruit. Not to mention that Maria was so generous to offer it to us, it would have been rude to pass it up! Let me tell you—it was the best mango I have ever had. We sat munching away, on the ground in the shade of the very tree the mango came from, and Maria began her story.

"My child was already ten months old when she died. We think it might have been malaria because she only had a fever."

At that point, Maria was already a mother of four little ones, her first three with a two-year spread between each of them. Later, far after the death of her little one, she would have three more—another girl and a set of twins.

"It was a Sunday, and the facility only takes emergencies on Sundays. I didn't know that this was an emergency." Maria looked away, the sequins on her black headscarf catching little rays of sunlight that filtered through the trees.

Maternal and infant health goes further than safe pregnancies or unattended childbirth. The more women I spoke to, and the more time I spent understanding the families and their struggles, the more I realized the depth of the problem.

There is never one solution or one cause to a crisis. When a mama loses her child, when Maria lost her ten-month-old little girl, there were a hundred factors that could contribute to the death. The cause could be as simple as the mosquito that carried the malaria—without which the little one wouldn't have been infected in the first place. Or, it could be the lack of accessible care, or the disparity of knowledge on the subject. It could be any number of reasons or all of them combined.

I looked into Maria's face, and I realized that in this moment, her situation, her geographical location, her level of education—none of it mattered. What mattered was that her child had died. The tiny girl whom she had fed, washed, and watched grow. Had she had the chance to say her first word? Toddle her first little steps? Understand the undying love her mama had for her?

"I never expected that my child would die," Maria looked at Agness as she spoke. It was painful for me to hear her words, even when they were filtered through a translator.

Agness pointed in the direction of a little clump of trees. It was the one place in the visible village that seemed to be left alone—unused and untamed. "There's two graveyards in most villages. One is the adult cemetery, where they bury most of their community. Then there is the child cemetery. Infants who have died under four months are buried there."

"Maria's daughter was ten months old when she died," I stared at the tiny stones that I could see peeking over the long grass. "Does that mean she would be buried in the adult graveyard?"

Agness nodded, after confirming it with Maria. It seemed strange that there would be a segregated cemetery specifically for infants. Were they less important? I didn't understand it completely but realized that the Malawian culture existed with a more developed appreciation and acceptance of infant mortality. Though never anticipated, it was more accepted and understood than the culture in which I had been raised.

Maria is one of hundreds of mothers who have lost their little ones in Malawi. She's one of hundreds of mamas who have had to prematurely bury their children. I was speaking to this with my dad a few days later, and he keenly observed something that I had missed.

He likened it to car accidents in North America. Though devastating, and variably impactful, we all know at least one person who's been in an accident. But we accept it because it's just a part of life. When maternal and infant mortality is as high as it is in Malawi, they are inevitably better trained to accept it. Everyone knows at least one mama who has lost a child.

Death in Malawi, though devastating and variably impactful, almost becomes just another part of life.

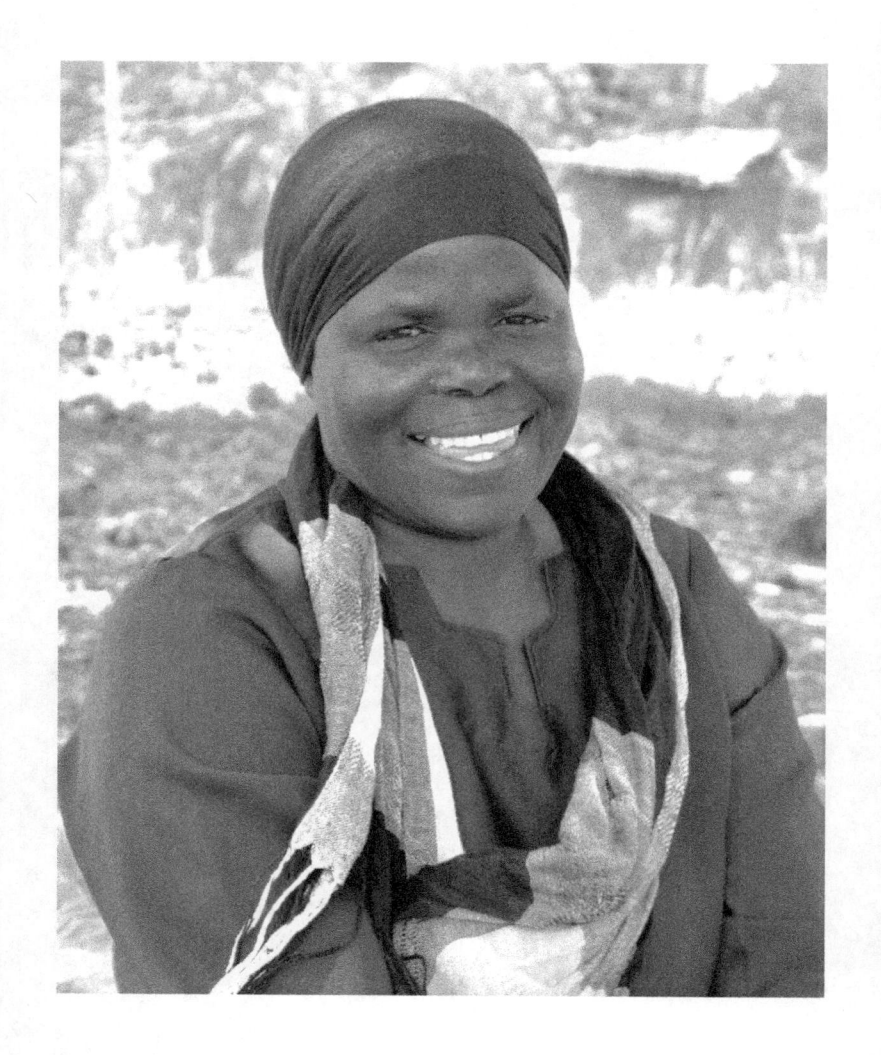

KATHERINE

I spoke with three mamas that day. Fynes and Maria, whom you have already met, and Katherine, whose words have reverberated through my mind most often. She was only twenty-one years old when she lost her child.[*] It was her very first one.

Though the event took place eighteen years ago, Katherine explained that she fully understood the harsh realities of her situation. "I had to accept what happened. I still wanted more children, though I waited a few years."

She was a strong woman who, despite her tragedy, learned to speak freely of her experience. Now, she's a mother of four children, and she often helps other mamas in her village process similar experiences.

"I might have contributed to the death of my child," Katherine's confession threw me completely off guard. Such a simple statement was drowning in years of hurt. My curious mind was begging to uncover the story, but my breaking heart knew I had to be gentle.

"What do you mean?" It was moments like these that I regretted our language barrier the most. Agness, my gift

---

[*] Her story impacts me in a unique way because at the time I spoke with her, I was also twenty-one years old.

from God, was a hundred times the translator and helper that I could have prayed for, but as Katherine began to share her story and I waited patiently for Agness's English to interrupt, I wished with all my heart that I could have understood the words firsthand.

"It was her first child," Agness said. "She didn't know much about the process of pregnancy and childbirth, though now she assures me that she has learned a lot." She continued, repeating Katherine's story to me.

"It was the middle of the night when I began labor. I was anemic, though I didn't know it yet. I had gone to see the doctor once before, when I was five months pregnant. I didn't know the dangers of only going once."

This was something that I had been hearing more about throughout my time in Malawi. When we first visited Bimbi Health Facility, Agness explained to me their initiatives to encourage more women to come for checkups throughout the duration of their pregnancy. The concept of regular checkups was uncommon to many Malawians, even nurses and midwives were being refreshed on basic check-up practices and effective ways to encourage more mothers to come for prenatal care.

When I spoke to Anke, the German gynecologist, she expressed shock and concern to me, explaining an encounter she had earlier that week. A mama in the hospital where she was volunteering had died earlier because of severe blood loss. When Anke checked into her records, she was surprised to see that this woman had been into the scheduled prenatal appointments. Digging a little deeper, Anke discovered that out of the five times the expectant mother had visited, her blood pressure had only been taken once.

"They are supposed to check blood pressure every single time. As often as they can," Anke's German accent couldn't hide the urgency she felt. "If she had been properly monitored, they would have known the mother was anemic. They could have prepared in advance. They would have been able to easily save her life."

In the same way, that was how Katherine discovered that she was also anemic. In the deep pains of heavy labor. In the dizzying swirl of blood loss. She was able to receive a blood transfusion when she finally reached the hospital, but by then it was too late for her child.

"I wasn't listening closely to the doctor either," Katherine continued. "I would be pushing when I wasn't supposed to be. He would tell me to stop pushing, to wait a little longer. But I didn't listen to him."

The baby was born without the ability to breathe on its own. A short three hours after she entered the world, Katherine's little one was lost.

"It was really painful for me," The heavy weight of death pronouncing itself in Katherine's voice. "I was never able to breastfeed her. I was never able to watch her grow."

In all my dreams of raising my kids, all the pleasures that come when a new mother first lays her eyes on her beautiful child, all of the unquenchable love and inconceivable joy that fills her when the little one is placed into her arms the first time—I couldn't possibly fathom what pain Katherine (and so many other mamas) must have felt when the little life was closed and stilled forever.

Katherine developed a severe case of pneumonia immediately following the delivery and was kept in the hospital for a month afterward. Three years later, she gave birth to her second child, who she was able to watch grow and flourish into the strong fifteen-year-old they are today.

With Agness's help and steady compassion, I was able to see the beacon of hope that is shimmering bright for mamas all throughout Malawi. This woman, alongside so many more, has suffered the painful outcome of poor maternal health. She's seen and experienced firsthand the cause and effect; the lack of accessible health care, the limited education, the genuine ignorance all factored into the death of her little one.

But Katherine is also the mother to four more children. She is a statistic, but a statistic of hope—a number that shows the ever-increasing rise of health. She is proof that maternal and infant mortality is a conquerable epidemic—a battle that ends with victory.

Our driver was delayed in returning to the village to pick up Agness and I again, so we sat on our thin straw mat underneath the trees to wait. For our conversation, Agness, Katherine, and I had been alone, but as the tone changed, several other mamas within the village joined us.

I sat silently in the filtered sunlight, watching the women laugh and chat with each other. Our little straw mat carried a joyful population of nearly ten women, their children of various ages running about.

A tiny little girl in a faded yellow dress bounced on her mother's lap. A three-year-old son played with a mango pit just to the side of me. Agness made a joke as a little one fussed against his mother's breast, and our company laughed, sparking the Chichewa conversation to roll forward.

I watched Katherine too. The way she smiled, the glow

of her eyes, rich in joy and love. Does Katherine see her unknown child in any of these little faces? Even after eighteen years, does she watch other children grow, imagining what the face of the little one who only lived three hours would have looked like today? Yet as I watched her laugh and smile with the other mamas, my heart sang praises to the hope and happiness she emanated.

I never expected hope like this to come out of something as tragic as an infant's death. I know it took Katherine many years to overcome the pain. You can still hear it in her voice when she talks of her lost little one. But Katherine has also had the joy of raising several more children; in the wake of tragedy hope remains. In fact, hope flourishes.

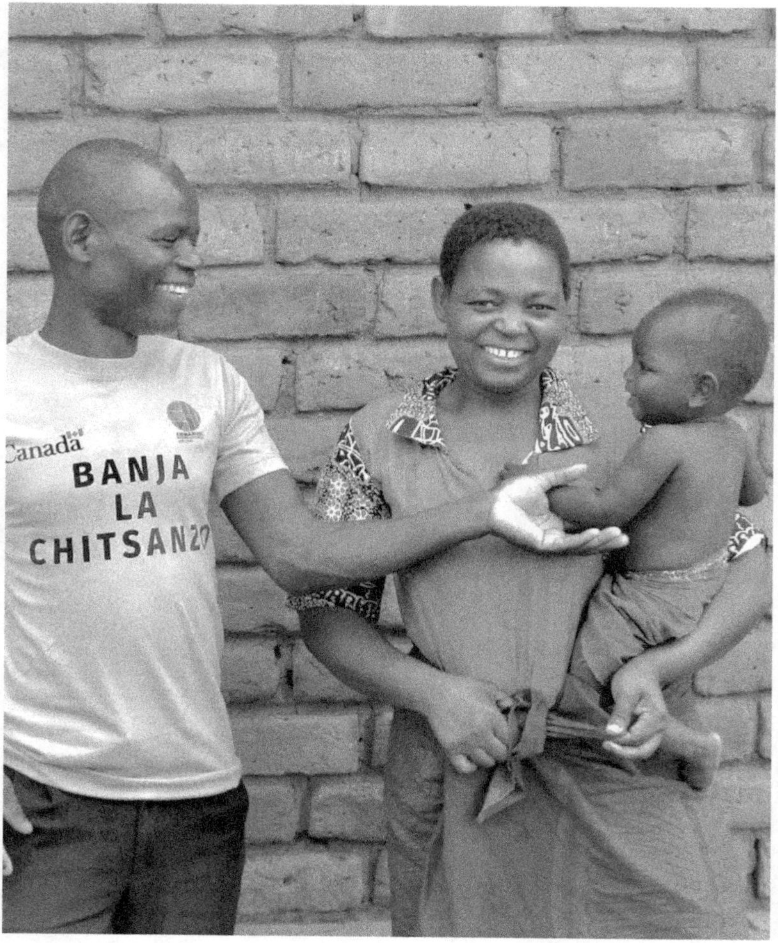
Canada
BANJA
LA
CHITSANZ?

MR. AND MRS. MCHENGA

I may have been mistaken in an earlier chapter of this book. In my defense, it was written before I met with Mr. and Mrs. Mchenga of Bimbi village, and no fortune teller could have predicted the information they shared with me.

My mistake lies in the bold statement when I shared the story of Francis: *I decided this was to be one of my favorite interviews.* Granted, every member of this collection was wonderful to meet. Every mama, nurse, child, and expert I have consulted were valuable, stimulating, and possessive of a very soft place in my heart. But the day I met Mr. and Mrs. Mchenga is one of my favorite stories to share simply because of the absolute treasure they are to each other, their five children, and the whole village surrounding them.

I had actually spoken with three couples in the span of that sun-baked afternoon, each of them just as inspirational as the next. The absolute joy and love that filled my conversations that afternoon is so strong that it seeps into every retelling of the story.

We were originally seated under a tree much closer to the main road, but we had barely begun our conversation before Agness interrupted, "I think we should move ourselves somewhere a bit more private." A little group of listeners had begun to gather, curious of what we wanted with their favored couple. I laughed in agreement, knowing the topic of our conversation might be easier said without the rest of the village in attendance.

Someone called out in Chichewa, an obvious taunt and jest, causing the Mchengas to laugh and throw their hands up. It was a rickety, time-worn bench that leaned against the side of a red-brick house where we eventually settled. I'm not confident which of the three couples actually lived in that house—if any of them at all—but it was of no consequence. The ground had absolutely no grass on it, but the dusty yard was swept and clean, its color matching the bricks of the building. We sat in the shade of the wall, close enough to the main road that the couple's friends would call to them as they walked or rode past on bicycles. They would raise their hand back, calling out in response to their friends, laughing before returning to our conversation.

A common theme of relationship-building, gender equality, and shared responsibilities in family care ran throughout almost all of my conversations in this book. Eventually, Agness and I decided it would make the most sense to talk to a few couples who had figured out ways to make it work, and who were also passing the knowledge on to other couples in the village.

The health of a marriage is significantly linked to the health of a mother and child. Though this may be a straightforward concept, seeing it exemplified so strongly on this short afternoon was inspiring. It is undeniable the impact that growing love and ongoing communication meant to these couples, their children, and any of their relationships.

Mr. and Mrs. Mchenga were of those three couples that I spoke with. They carried with them their youngest child, a five-month swaddle of white crocheted blankets and blue knitted hats. I was barely able to make out a face through all that cloth.

"Tell me your story," I began, excited to discover the foundation of the obvious joy the couple shared. "How did you two meet?"

I was absolutely thrilled with their answer.

It had been a normal day for the both of them. There was no event, no significant reason that they would be walking down the road that day. But it so happens that under the sunshine and on the red dust roads, the two of them coincidentally crossed paths. He was walking towards the village; she was walking away from it.

They didn't tell me the exact words that they greeted each other with, but the heavens must have sung, and light must have fallen upon them, because three months after they met on the road, they had married.

"Three months!" When you know, you know, I suppose. "What made you decide to get married so soon?"

She laughed at him, her eyes glinting, "Well honestly, my husband just wanted to! He asked, and I thought, why not? Of course, I said yes!"

"I'll tell you," Her husband interrupted her, his thin arms bouncing the bundle of blankets up and down. "Those first days of our marriage were really, really nice. But now, they're even nicer!"

She laughed and chastised him in Chichewa for a moment. His smile displaced the silver stubble of his beard. "Of course, it wasn't always nice. Sometimes it was quite difficult. Sometimes my wife would not be home for a long period of time, so we would argue because of that."

But there were traditional marriage counselors around who taught them etiquette tips for how to treat each other, how to manage money, how to be honest with their spouse.

The Makupes were another couple that I spoke with that day. They sat on the same bench and relayed similar issues that they had in their six years of marriage.

"For me it was quite difficult," Mr. Makupe told me. "I wasn't financially stable or ready for marriage. It was our parents who really made us get married."

Mrs. Makupe is one of the several members of the Gender Committee in Bimbi village. The Committee was formed and supported by the maternal health program. Essentially, it is meant to integrate a stronger notion of gender equality, male involvement in the family, and strong marriage values throughout the village.

Traditionally and culturally, there is a divide between men and women. Quite often, fathers are less involved with family life and less communicative in a marriage. Infidelity is all too common, leading to an unhealthy distrust between a couple. Their finances become secretive and eventually what once was a loving partnership falls apart.

According to USAID, "Women and girls in Malawi fare worse than their male counterparts on socio-economic indicators including literacy, secondary and tertiary education enrolment and completion, wage equality, [and] political participation. And, while an adequate legal framework exists, the public and non-governmental sector responses to gender-based violence are under-resourced, uncoordinated, and inadequate."[xv]

It's an ever-present problem within Malawian households, this concept of Gender Based Violence. It doesn't just cover physical abuse as the name suggests but is a term that is meant to address gender equality and the overall fair treatment of women within Malawi.

Agness, my constant source of knowledge, explained how their program worked to integrate marital health with maternal health and how the effects of it were undeniably positive. "Members of the Gender Committee and the Health Care Promoters will offer training for couples in their villages."

These groups were already formed by a previous government initiative, so when the new maternal health program entered, it was surprisingly easy to find the manpower required to carry out their initiatives. As the program became increasingly successful, the committees grew.

"The program encourages things like communication, working together and openness in a marriage. We also encourage men to be more involved with the prenatal process, asking them to come with their wives during their routine visits. The healthier a marriage, the healthier the mother and child are," Agness reiterated.

Mr. and Mrs. Makaika have seen the immediate impact of the program, noting just how much it helped their marriage and children. "Before, we weren't really communicating well. We were always fighting. I wasn't being very transparent about income either," Mr. Makaika admitted.

He looked at me when he spoke, though I could only understand his words through Agness's translation. His deep voice matched the hushed tones of the wind through the leaves of the baobab tree and bamboo bush that we sat next to. The man was strong, his muscles barely covered by the program t-shirt that he wore. But his face was gentle and kind. It had a handsome element that reflected a deep character and genuine passion.

"But now we're being open with each other. We're more romantic. We share our feelings, and we stop holding grudges."

His wife smiled at him, adding, "At first it seemed we were going our separate ways. But we elected to attend the training and things really improved. Our children are living free, they're healthy too!"

"What do you do to make sure you're always communicating?" I asked, curious to see their strategies. "Do you have any examples?"

"Sometimes you hear a rumour about your spouse," Mrs. Makaika began. "They tell you, 'they were here at this time,' or 'they went out with so-and-so.' But the trick is to just not believe it. You go straight to your spouse and ask them. Be open about it."

"We also work side by side to have a good garden," her husband added. "I will dig the ground, and my wife takes away the weeds. We plant the seeds together."

All of the couples that Agness and I met that day were playful and full of laughter. They joked with each other and with Agness and me. The light in their eyes shone brighter when they talked of their love for each other—the way they've learned to communicate and work together and lead other couples to be just as strong.

We were wrapping up our conversation with Mr. and Mrs. Mchenga, regretfully watching the sun hover dangerously close to the horizon. The man, with his beard and knobbly hands bouncing the massive bundle of blankets around the baby on his lap looked prouder than ever to be sitting exactly where he was.

"Before we go," I started, anxious to have more time with this jovial couple. "Tell me this. After fifteen years of marriage, you'll know each other so well. What is one thing that you love most about each other?"

I didn't ask either one in particular, but Mr. Mchenga was quick to answer. The vision of his wife's shocked face, and the three's abrupt laughter is a moment that I will always be able to replay in my mind. I had to wait for Agness and the couple to compose themselves before I could be let in on the joke, but it all made sense the second Agness turned to me.

She clasped her hands on her knees, intentionally avoiding my eyes. "He said, 'My favorite thing? After all these years, she's still very good in bed.'"

The three of them laughed again as I turned red, my mouth reactively falling open.

Mrs. Mchenga pushed her husband, rocking the unstable bench. But she was blushing, her grand eyes full of happiness.

As we departed, I soaked in the warm wind waving the trees and carrying us home. The sun sank below the two peaks of the Zomba mountain, and the pleasure of the day welled in my heart.

Where there is love, there is hope; where there is hope, there is joy. I felt joy within these Malawian couples all day—their lives full of hope and the promise of bright futures together.

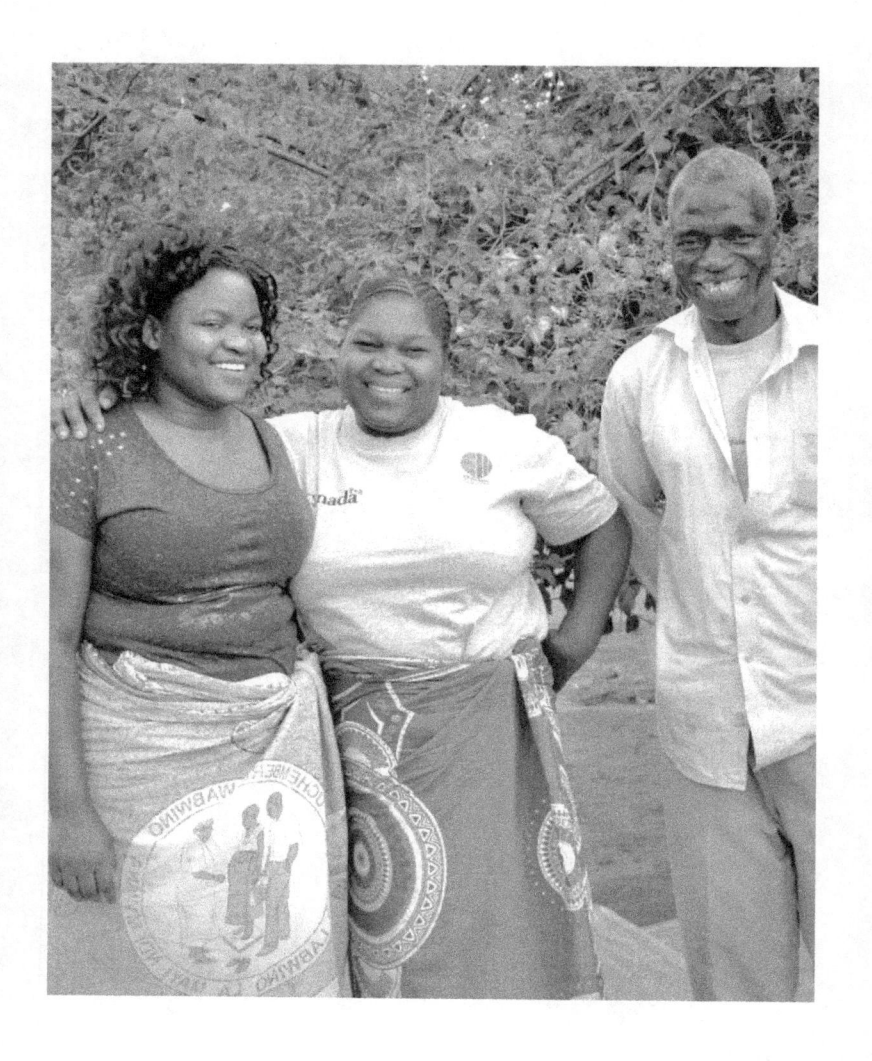

DYSON AND ESNAT

Driving farther into the villages and away from the main road felt like someone was slowly putting a sepia filter on the landscape. The dusty brown seemed to creep from the unpaved roads and onto the trees, fields, grass, and mountains. Even the sky seemed to be a hazy brown. It made for a fascinating canvas of deeper and lighter tones of the reddish-brown paint that seemed to have so delicately spread out over the world.

There was, however, my favorite exception.

Every so often, as we would drive or walk the sepia roads, a brilliant glow of color would shine like a beacon in the nighttime sea. In the middle of a village, the center of a field, perched on the side of the road; there were little gifts of the sun in the form of the brightest flowering trees.

The trees aren't the blush-pink or soft white of the crab apples or magnolia trees that bloom in Canadian springtime. Far from it. Their seasoned petals donned colors of neon orange, rich fuchsias, and deep purples. Malawi is home to trees that flower year-round, and while you can go out at any moment to see the blossoms, they strike you the hardest when it's the only flash of color on a wide, sepia horizon. They are unmistakable and simply breathtaking.

I spent an entire afternoon under one of such trees, its pure magenta petals as large as its leaves offered a breathtaking backdrop to the conversation I was having with Dyson and Esnat. Interestingly, I hadn't come to hear their stories.

They were Health Promoters, and Agnes knew them from her work in the village. Word must have spread quickly about our arrival because before long, Agness and I had an audience. Dyson and Esnat had been watching us from a short distance; when we said farewell to the women we had originally been sitting with, they came quickly to greet us.

They chatted for a while, catching each other up on the project progress while I waited, mesmerized under the magenta tree. At one point, Agness turned to introduce us, asking, "Do you want me to translate for them too?"

"Of course!" I told her; saying *no* to a conversation went against every grain of extroverted fiber in my body. It was a good thing that I did too.

Health Promoters, as we've seen, are influential members of their communities and villages. They're part of care groups that are established to help guide the communities toward greater health practices including hygiene, nutrition, and knowledge empowerment.

Dyson and Esnat took the place of the women I had just been chatting with and seated themselves gracefully on the straw mat underneath the neon petals. We settled in and I began peppering them with improvised questions—wanting to understand every element of their tasks, their goals for the communities, and their own stories as they work together.

"Have seen much change in your villages, then?" I

asked, following their descriptions of the tasks and duties they have as Health Promoters. I didn't have to wait for Agness's translation of their answer; it was written clearly on their faces.

"Of course!" Agness's voice repeated Dyson's response. "Our groups give us training to help us be more effective, and it's really working! So many habits have changed. Hygiene, nutrition, and, of course, empowering women by reducing the knowledge gap."

"What do you mean by that?" I asked, scribbling down the term in my blue spiral notepad. "What is the 'knowledge gap'?"

It was, as I learned, a contribution to the inequality within households between men and women. It manifested itself in feelings of superiority or inferiority when one member of a family had more education, or knowledge, than another. In Malawi, as it is in many other countries, thousands of women have less of an opportunity to attend school than their male counterparts. As a result, the knowledge gap often presents itself most significantly between men and women.

As we know, education is essential for empowerment. There have been studies that show that the more years spent in school, there are greater health outcomes for women and their communities. In fact, "each additional year a girl stays in school is associated with a 10% increase in wages, increased life expectancy, and reduced fertility." The statistics are disheartening, with a mere 38% of women having completed primary school. "For every 100 girls who begin Standard 1, only about three will enter into secondary education. Of those three, only one will enter university." [xvi]

"But things are changing," Dyson said. "We work as a group—as a team—to reach the community as a whole."

"And those who don't know are taught by their own peers. They teach each other," Esnat finished Dyson's thought. "The women talk to each other around the bore hole, and that's where they learn. When you educate a few, you can change an entire village."

Dyson and Esnat represented a massive group of Health Promoters in the region. They received specific training and were required to attend follow-up meetings throughout the years. Their tasks are multi-faceted with the ultimate goal of changing the lives within their communities.

The roots of maternal and newborn health in Malawi are not healthy. They haven't been cultivated properly and haven't been fed the right resources and information to help them grow as they should. A higher quality of life and a more hopeful future in a culture like Malawi's includes reaching deep into the ancient clay and altering the shape of its roots. Health Promoters like Dyson and Esnat carry with them a contagious desire to change things for the betterment of their people.

"It took some time to convince the community to listen to us. But once one family is convinced, it has a domino effect," Dyson explained. "For instance, when we began, it was usual that households would share toilets. There would often be as many as five houses sharing one toilet!"

Agness looked at me with patient eyes; the surprise must have been written all over my face. I grew up in a house of five. My parents bought a cozy little bungalow built on a behind-the-scenes road between a forest and a lake when they first married, and they've been in that house ever since. My family always got along really well, but there were times when my meager family of five could barely handle sharing the one bathroom in our house. Between the five of us, I remember racing inside to be the first one in the bathroom after a long road trip. I remember knocking on the door countless times when my brother was taking too long in the shower. Even though we made it work for us, I still couldn't imagine having to share one toilet with not only my household but the next five homes on my street as well.

To be fair, bathroom habits in the villages of Malawi are generally very different than ours. Their toilets are made most often of mere holes in the ground, with a small corn-stalk enclosure to offer a little piece of privacy. I had learned of a movement that has been making its way through the country that encouraged concrete molds to cover the latrine hole, making it easier to clean and cover up as the hole filled. Sealing it with cement also offered a substantially less risk for contamination for those using the toilets.

The program Dyson, Esnat, and Agness are a part of also encourages a contraption they call 'tippy-taps' constructed of a supporting stick and filled water bottle. It serves as a hand-washing station for the latrine, offering an immediate place for toilet users to wash their hands once they're done.

"Just the simple act of rinsing your hands after using the toilet has significantly reduced disease and sickness throughout the villages," Agness told me, echoing what I've heard from many people prior to our conversation here. It prevents the bacteria from going any farther and spreading immeasurably to the people. When as many as five large families are sharing one latrine, you can be sure that their bacteria have an ever-increasing risk of spreading and infecting the community.

Esnat proudly offered the details of their victories, "It took us a little while, but now, out of the two communities we work with, nearly all of them have their own toilet. In one, all 108 houses have their own. Our second village was trickier. Of all 128 households, there are still three who are too stubborn to build one for themselves." She pursed her lips and tilted her head, "They'll come around, though."

"Is it always so difficult to convince people to practice new methods?" I asked the two of them.

Dyson nodded, "Sometimes it's very challenging. We will often volunteer our own resources to change a family or to support their kids."

I looked at them—their faces shining under the fuchsia petals—and I was unsurprised by their generosity. Impressed, but unsurprised. Dyson and Esnat were only two of many Health Promoters that I met throughout my stay, and many of them share the same qualities. Like Agness, they have an honest and genuine desire to see change in their people. They volunteer their time and fund certain elements with their own resources, learning, training, and traveling from door to door to promote healthier living.

As the two left to finish their day, I considered the comparison of a single-colored life, swirls of bright hues being thrown in to act as beacons of hope. The cause-and-effect cycle and consequences of poor maternal health are numerous. The more I dig into it, the deeper it seems. But here are people, like the bright trees in the landscape, who offer a promise of hope and change in a way that not many can.

With that in mind, Agness and I waited happily under the fluorescent petals for our white truck to come and pick us up, taking us back home through a cloud of sepia dust.

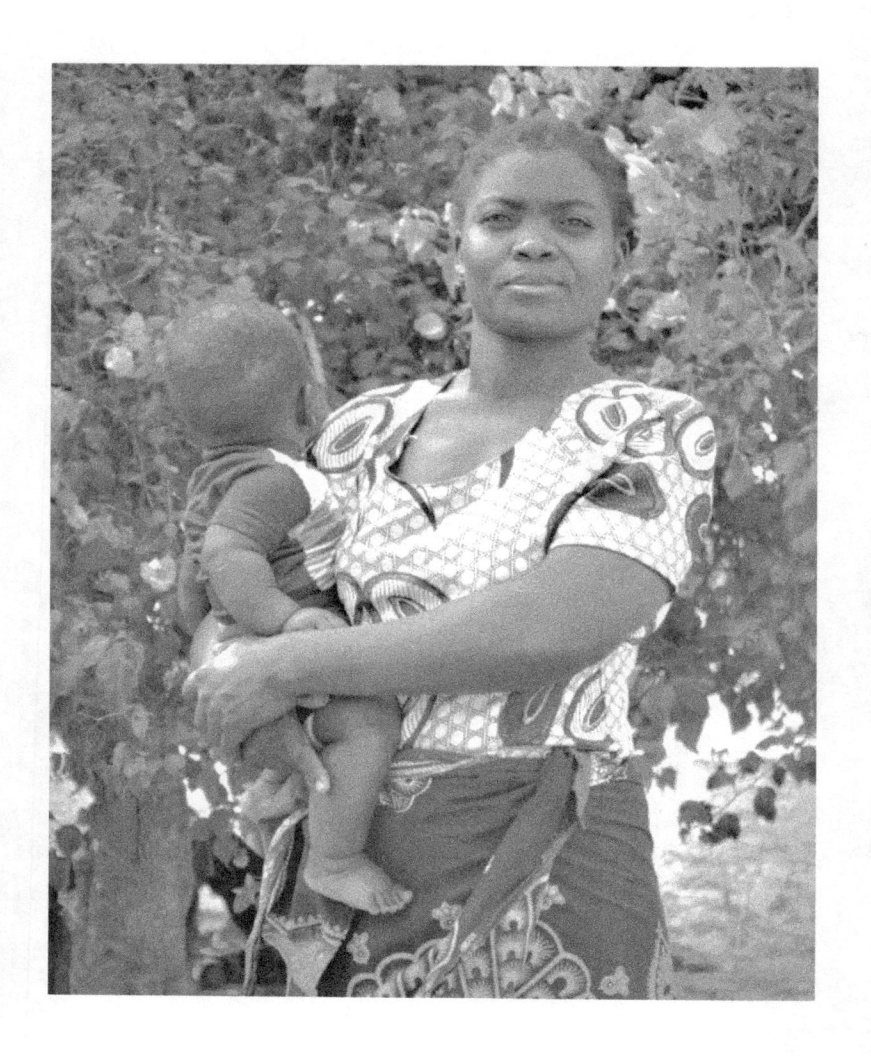

GERTRUDE

"Being alone isn't easy. Sometimes I still go hungry."

I was chatting with Gertrude on a mat made from dried grass and flour sacks under the same flowering tree that I met Dyson and Esnat previously.

As always, the village must have been made aware that Agness and I were on our way, because the large woven mat placed on top of the dirt before we had arrived, accompanied by two tiny chairs that wobbled on the uneven ground. If there was ever a stool to sit on, the hosts would often insist that Agness and I take it—even if whomever it was that I was speaking with were much older or seemingly more fragile than myself.

Such was the case with Gertrude—a stout woman somewhere in her mid-fifties. She didn't present herself as someone unable to sit lower on the thin woven mat, but it went against my raising to be sitting on an elevated spot when my host had to take the floor. I always perched myself lightly on the edge when my trip first began, uncomfortable and ready to offer it away at a moment's notice. But Agness taught me that it was more respectful to accept the worn wooden chairs than to refuse, and it slowly became easier to relax.

By the time I spoke with Gertrude, I was more than

aware of the multi-layered issue that maternal health in Malawi is, and how it individually manifests itself within different lives. More than the 'basic' reduction of death and injury to mothers and children, the problem stems outward in all directions—one of the branches reaching through the doors and into the home. It manifests itself in the treatment and respect of women.

I told Agness that I wanted to speak with someone like Gertrude. I wanted to understand life from the perspective of someone whose experiences are like hers. When Agness introduced me to Gertrude, I was impressed all over again with the perseverance and strength that the people in this country hold so deeply within themselves.

The woman sitting before me on the mat with her legs outstretched before her had been married for sixteen years. She had six children with her husband, the youngest of which was only five months old at the time I spoke with her. I realized that she would have carried the youngest little one all alone, having divorced her husband only a year before we met.

She may not have even known she was pregnant until after the divorce.

"Tell me about it," I prompted. "After sixteen years, why separate now?"

"It was a matter of gender-based violence." Curls on Agness's head bounced around her shoulders as she translated. "He was abusive. He was unfaithful. He was stealing our money for himself."

My heart broke. I had heard that story before, described in a similar way by other mothers I spoke with. Gertrude's story was uniquely painful to her and her children, but not at all unheard of.

"I was there for sixteen years, and I tried to make a change. We even tried to see village counselors. But he wasn't going to be changing, I knew that."

I tried to interpret the expression Gertrude held on her face. Many Malawian women that I met carried themselves with upright resolve. At times, a glimpse of resignation could be seen through the keyhole into their lives that I looked through.

Gertrude's face seemed to carry a different story. She was tired. Her posture as she sat beneath the pink petals, protected by the thin mat from the dust below, was a clear expression of weariness. She was tired of the pain, tired of the hunger, tired of feeling trapped.

"But then, what do you do?" I asked, pausing to let Agness interpret. "How are you able to support your children?"

"I sell *mandasi*," she responded, Agness explaining a little bit further, "You know those deep-fried dough that you see being sold on the road all the time? That's *mandasi*. They're like doughnuts, only less sweet."

If you were to take any road in Malawi, you are sure to see multiple vendors carrying their fresh batches of *mandasi* in their sealed buckets—balanced on their heads, calling in advertisement to the passers-by. It wasn't just *mandasi* that you would see. In some of the more populous villages near the main road, there would be vendors selling grilled maize, popped corn, or similar treats. They were sold by every demographic. Mothers, children, fathers—they all had a place selling what they could to those in the villages.

"My older children will often come and take care of the kids too," Gertrude smiled.

Another woman I asked about being a single mother emphasized how lonely it was. "My heart beats for a man," she described poetically, a hand to her chest for emphasis.

Being a single parent in Canada has its own associated struggles and pains, and Gertrude's story parallels many of the struggles that exist in the single parents I know. But her story also exposes the additional weight and struggle that a single mother in Malawi must endure.

Maternal health is so much more than pregnancy and childbearing. It extends to healthy relationships and the general care of women. The maternal health program has a massive emphasis on healthy relationships on top of proper breastfeeding and nutrition practices. As we've already seen, the villages are taught the importance of strong communication between couples, and how to be open and honest with each other. They're taught how to work together and respect each other, allowing for the best health of the family, including the mothers and children. A healthy marriage will lead to a healthier lifestyle, better nutrition, greater access to health care, and the overall preservation of lives.

"I have learned what a marriage should look like," Gertrude told me. She had participated in the Healthy Relationship workshops in the village. "And I'm raising my children to see the difference."

Admittedly, life is much different for her now without a husband. She has no second source of income and no helper when she needs one. "I would marry again," Gertrude said, clasping her hands shyly in her lap. "But only if I find the right suitor."

For now, despite the added concerns of single-handedly providing for six children and herself, Gertrude is away from the abuse. She's protected from the lying and cheating, the stealing and beating. She has the opportunity to learn about how to care for herself and lead a healthier life, providing the right nutrition for her kids, particularly her brand new little one.

"How can you be sure you've made the right choice?" I asked, referencing all the difficulties of single parenthood, particularly those unique to her situation.

Gertrude closed her tired eyes and bowed her head toward her lap. But her face was smiling.

"I just wanted to be free."

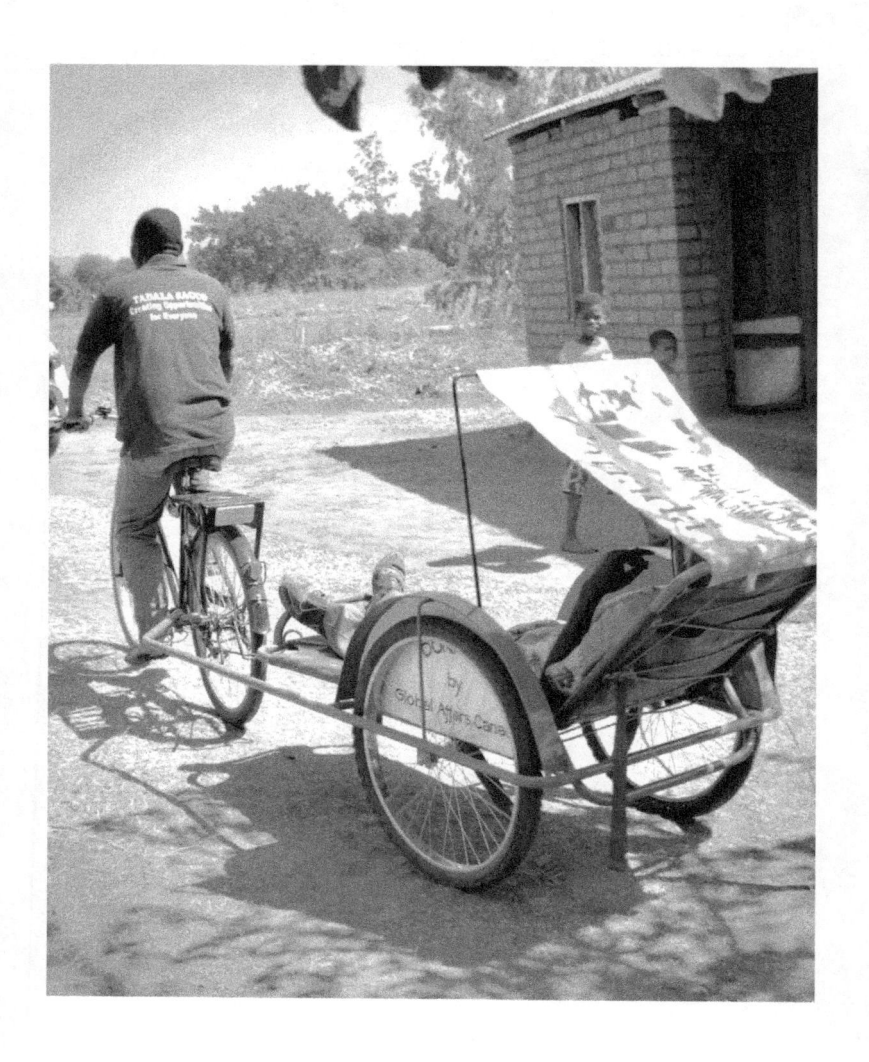

DECEMBER

The day I met Kevin was very hot.

I can't remember feeling uncomfortably hot, but that's not surprising given my love for summertime. However, I know that the sun was strong and the earth was radiating because I have a distinct memory of the little beads of sweat on the foreheads of the crowd around us. I can envision Agness taking the corner of her bright blue *chitenge* and patting the sweat off of her upper lip.

But I don't mind the heat, so I let my eyes bounce back and forth, capturing everything in my mind as personal treasures.

Our driver dropped us off by the village well, which was currently in use by several women and their children. The mothers chatted in the shade while the kids heaved the pump up and down. There were a few free-range chickens playing in one of the puddles that tricked down from the well's off spout.

They waved and called out to Agness and I as we passed, starting our ten-minute trek down the road towards the place we would meet Kevin. It was someone else's crude brick home, with a rare tin roof.

We rarely entered anyone's house, as meeting outdoors was often easier and allowed for a fresh breeze to accompany our conversation. But on this rare occasion, our hosts invited us inside for a moment as we waited for Kevin and the others to arrive.

This home belonged to one of the village leaders. It had four rooms; the front entrance, and three others that I assumed served as bedrooms. There were no doors in the door frames, no glass in the windows, and the dirt floors were more or less void of the furniture and décor I was used to seeing back home. I shouldn't have been surprised—Malawians spend most of their days outside, so it would make sense that their homes wouldn't collect the same kind of clutter and possessions that your typical North American household would. Regardless, it felt strange that the plastic chairs in the room were the same we sat on outdoors and would be returned to their places beneath the tree once we left.

Not every home was as empty as this one. Depending on the wealth or culture of the village, some homes carried bigger beds, mosquito nets and decorative curtains. I could tell that this home was not standard for this particular village, so I made a mental note to appreciate it.

Agness and I sat in their home, chatting with the homeowner and his wife as we waited. He spoke a fair amount of English, so the four of us were able to have an easier conversation without the need for Agness's translation skills. The couple teased me about being from Canada, asking me to describe the snow and the landscapes and how different it is from Malawi. They were shocked when I told them how much I loved the heat in Malawi, and nearly cried when I told them it was a nice escape from the -30 degrees Celsius we were about to endure in the Canadian winter.

Kevin arrived with an entourage, several men with curious energy, wanting to know why I wanted to speak with Kevin, what Agness and a mysterious *mzungu* were doing in their village.

They were able to play their part far sooner than any of us expected, as we discovered that one of the men was the keeper of the village bicycle ambulance.

He introduced himself to me as December, and he was equally thrilled to show me as I was to see the bicycle ambulance on display. The men hurried with excitement to show me how it worked, each one anxious to describe how the carrier connected to the bike and how the sun-shelter assembled so quickly.

The bike was donated by the PROMISE organization and brought to the village as a cost-effective and adaptable method of transportation for women in labor (and all other kinds of emergencies) to the Bimbi Health Facility.

"We use it almost once a week," December explained as he pulled its components together. "We have had a number of cases where the men were sick or unconscious, but we made it to the hospital on time to help them and save their lives."

December and his friends demonstrated how these ambulances were so much more effective than before. Their village, being incredibly far from the main road, meant that it took nearly an hour to reach the clinic on a good day. To extend the problem, a regular ambulance would have greater difficulty blazing through the village footpaths, which were not designed for a motorized vehicle in any way. Depending on the village, it could sometimes take anywhere up to five hours for an ambulance to arrive.

The bicycle ambulance was actually more of a cart that was secured behind a normal bicycle. Welded together by workers in the Malawi's Blantyre City, the cart was long enough to carry a grown man, and just wide enough for a mother and child. The back was raised into a lounging position, and a detachable sunshade was positioned overtop.

I watched, laughing as the group of men argued who would sit in the cart, and who would pedal the bike in order to demonstrate how it worked. Eventually, one of them threw themselves on the bicycle ambulance and December took off as the driver, leaving an echo of laughter behind them in the dust.

"We got our second bicycle ambulance two months ago," December said when they finally returned on the bike. "But our area is so large—it has to serve ours and the next village over."

A total of thirty-six bicycle ambulances had been distributed to over thirteen villages, but it was, of course, never enough.

"How often would you say you take women in labor?" I thought back to my friend Maria, who had delivered and lost her little one on the side of the road because there was nothing like this available for her in her village.

December's face fell for a moment. "We haven't taken many women yet. When they're in labor, they don't often want many people to know. So, they will only call us to take them to the clinic when something goes really wrong."

By then, I thought, it's almost too late.

"Things are changing, though," December assured me, confidence strengthening his voice. "Things are going to improve."

The culture of motherhood was shifting. More women were learning about the importance of visiting the clinic and birthing there too. They were learning to care for themselves and their children in brand new ways, breaking an unhealthy cycle of misinformation and unhealthy practices. Though sometimes resistant to change, seeing its effectiveness was always the greatest push.

December was confident in the progress, the shift in maternal health culture, and was honored to be part of it. We spoke some more about the benefits of traveling by bicycle and the need for more of such ambulances to be donated to the villages, and I hastened to jot down the stories that December and his cohort shared.

But there was someone present whose experience I particularly wanted to know more about, and so finally, after very patiently waiting, I turned to Kevin.

"Tell me your story," I said.

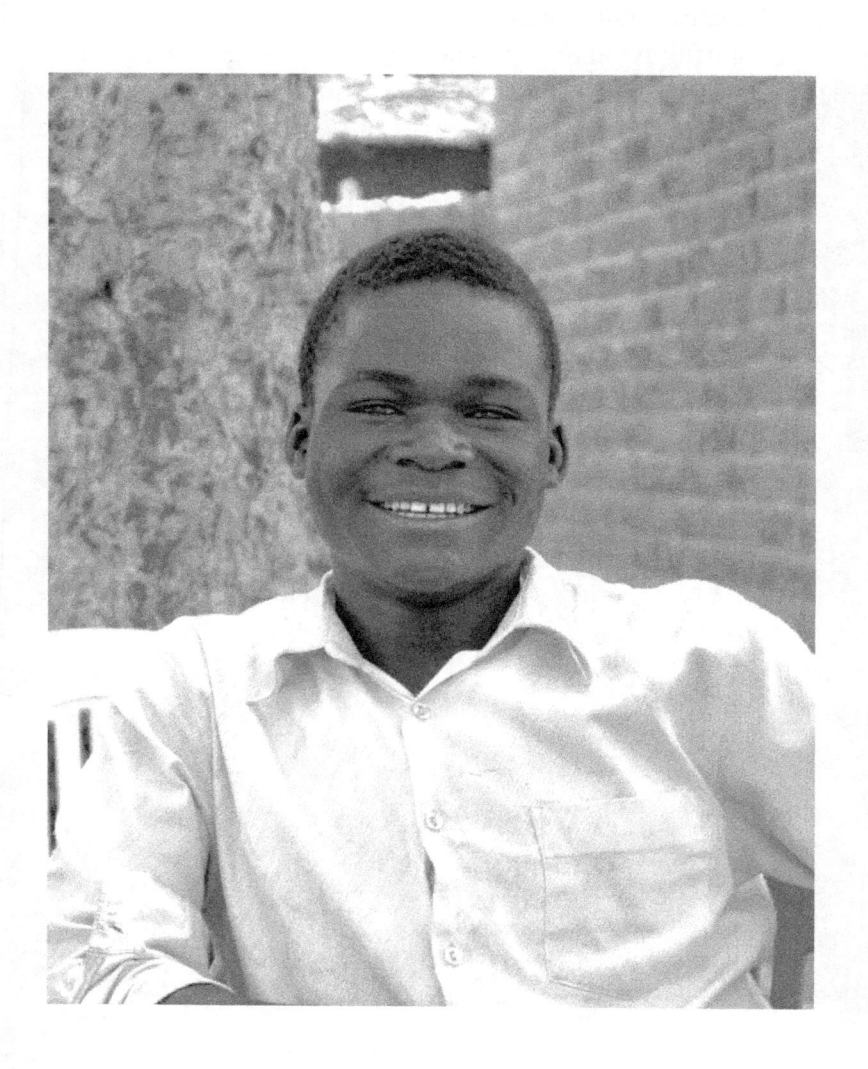

KEVIN

Kevin was definitely not fifteen years old.

He was, but I could hardly believe it. Even Agness said to me afterwards, "Kevin seemed so much older than his age!"

I thought so too. To begin, he had the bone structure of a twenty-year-old. His body was strong, his shoulders broad and secure. His face held the calm wisdom and self-assurance that I had never before seen in a fifteen-year-old. I coveted it, wishing I could adopt his stoic stature for myself.

He was the kind of boy who fit in better with grown men like December than the boys his own age at school. He seemed to understand things far beyond what he should for someone his age. Even without all the prejudices and predeterminations of what a fifteen-year-old should be like, I was impressed. The boy-man before me was an inspiration.

When I first arrived in Malawi and met Agness, I gave her a list of the kinds of people I really wanted to meet with. Mothers, couples, nurses, and so forth would help me gain a complete and rounded understanding of maternal health in the area. I craved as many perspectives as possible in my limited timeline.

Agness was a true blessing from God, having organized all of her connections within two days, and Kevin was my little glimpse into the life of a young person. I asked Agness if she could introduce me to a young person, someone with siblings and parents and experience that was old enough to be influenced by goodness. Kevin was all these things and more.

He said hello to me in English and asked me how I was doing.

"I am doing well! How are you?" I smiled, impressed by his formal greeting.

The men had put their bicycle ambulance away and were sitting on the steps of the home, laughing.

"He doesn't speak English!" One of them called out in jest. Kevin blushed and shouted something back, sending them into a round of laughter again.[*]

Agness kicked things off properly, going through her regular introduction of who we were and what we were coming to talk about. Kevin nodded and introduced himself back to us.

"My name is Kevin. I'm fifteen. I have a sister too, who is seven."

"Tell me a little about you two! Do you get along?" I asked, Agness translated.

"Of course!" he smiled. "I have a good relationship with my sister. We take care of each other. She wants to be a teacher when she grows up."

---

[*] I liken this experience to my knowledge of French. Despite being Canadian and growing up taking French classes, I only know enough to answer a few questions at the grocery store or make a common greeting. I actually applied for a position once that required a bilingual candidate, and I completely botched the French part of the interview.

I scribbled down in my little blue notepad, "And what about you? Do you know what you'd like to be?"

Kevin's response was prompt. He knew exactly what he was striving for—and why. "I want to be a doctor. I have seen the way they work, and I want to be just like that. I know it's a lot of effort," he continued, "but I feel that if I work hard enough, and with God's help, I can achieve all these things."

The men waiting on the steps of the homestead were gently chatting amongst themselves. A goat from a nearby home wandered past, its chewed-through rope dangling inches above the ground. The air was hot and still. I wondered who it was that gave Kevin such confidence, and who it was that could help him continue to work and grow as he did. My questions lead me to what I really wanted to know; what the maternal health movement looked like to him, an aspiring doctor with mature, yet young eyes.

He thought for a moment when I asked him, then said, "It's really nice. At home, things are different."

"How so?"

It took me a while to figure out how to work through a translator to prompt out the kind of stories that I wanted to hear. People are a lot less open and talkative when they have to wait every few sentences for me to understand their words. But patience is a virtue, and with Agness's help, I nailed down a system that would often give me the depth of testimony that I desired. It's all in a matter of how you ask the question—and asking them in different ways.

He answered with a thoughtful response. "We didn't have the care or understanding of proper hygiene. We never used to wash our hands. Not before we ate or anything. But now we do. And there's no cholera at all."

There are no other transmittable diseases in the village either, Agness later told me. Apart from what comes through external forces, any disease that can be transmitted due to poor hygiene is nearly eradicated in Kevin's village.

"This program has helped our village in so many ways. They've provided us with the bicycle ambulance. They've taught us better hygiene. They've showed us the benefits of energy-saving stoves and helped us develop tippy-taps," He touched the tips of his fingers, counting the ways that he's helped contribute to these things as well—learning and watching how important they are to the health of the village and the health of the mothers.

I felt a foreign sense of pride for Kevin. Here was the boy whom I had known for all but half an hour, and yet I had observed his kindness, care, and wisdom that was far beyond his meager fifteen years of age—even culturally speaking. I was proud of him. Proud of the posture he held himself with on the plastic chair in the filtered shade. Proud of the deep insight he spoke with, equivalent to the men sitting on the dusty porch just behind him. Proud of the obvious quiet love he had for his sister and mother and village in which he lived. But what really moved me was the hope that Kevin carried with him.

I thought back to what Esnat the Health Promoter told me a few days prior. "When you educate a few, you can change an entire village." In other words, as little as one person can change the way an entire community approaches maternal health or anything, for that matter.

Kevin was a prime example of that. As he sees and grows excited about the great changes taking part in his community, he takes it with him throughout his life. He influences his peers and parents, friends and colleagues, pushing forward healthier, lifesaving practices. His seven-year-old sister will grow up in a village that doesn't see cholera. She, with her friends, will grow in a village with higher standards of nutrition, self-care, and respect for each other. The ripple effect of Kevin's life (and the individuals he is among) is the overall saving of mothers and children, men and their families. Kevin's influence has the opportunity to alter the culture of his entire village. I prayed that his zeal would never die.

Then Kevin continued, filling my heart completely. "The way I was thinking before has changed. It's changed for all of us."

Was this sweat in my eyes? Were they irritated from the dust in the air? I could have cried hearing Kevin's admission. The changing of the culture surrounding poor maternal health is entirely influenced by the way a community thinks. In Kevin's own words, the program has changed their mindsets. One by one, mothers and their vulnerable children will become stronger and healthier—their mortality risks lowering and dwindling altogether. My heart soared. The project was working, one village at a time.

I watched Kevin's manly front slip for a moment as Agness and I were preparing to leave. I thanked Kevin, expending my hand and clasping my wrist, as others did when they greeted me. A boyish grin fluttered across his face and he made a shy comment to Agness. She laughed, smacking his arm as he squirmed and pulled away. The men behind us who had heard the comment laughed as well.

"What did he say?" I asked, amused as he accepted my

outstretched hand and shook it.

"He wanted to say thanks for talking with him," Agness replied with a grin still on her cheeks. "But he said that it was weird talking to you, a *mzungu*. He said he had never spoken to one before."

"Well!" I said, amused, shocked, and a little flattered. "I hope I made a good impression. I wouldn't want to ruin it for the next *mzungu* he meets!"

Agness laughed again and relayed the message.

"I suppose other expats don't make it into their village very often?"

"We try to employ the locals as much as possible." There was a wink in her voice, confirming my thoughts.

I nodded, remembering the poor child who had burst into tears when I stepped out of the truck some time ago. I was likely the first *mzungu* the little two-year-old had ever seen, and she was clearly terrified by my presence. I would have been pretty shocked to see a pale, blonde-haired ghost at that age as well.

It didn't bother me that Kevin had made a comment about it. I knew it wouldn't make any difference to his approach. To his zeal. To his hope and outlook on life.

Kevin was an inspiration to his community and to me. This young man had the ability to take on an entire village and be a piece of the transformational work that is going on, and it was clear that he was ambitious to do so.

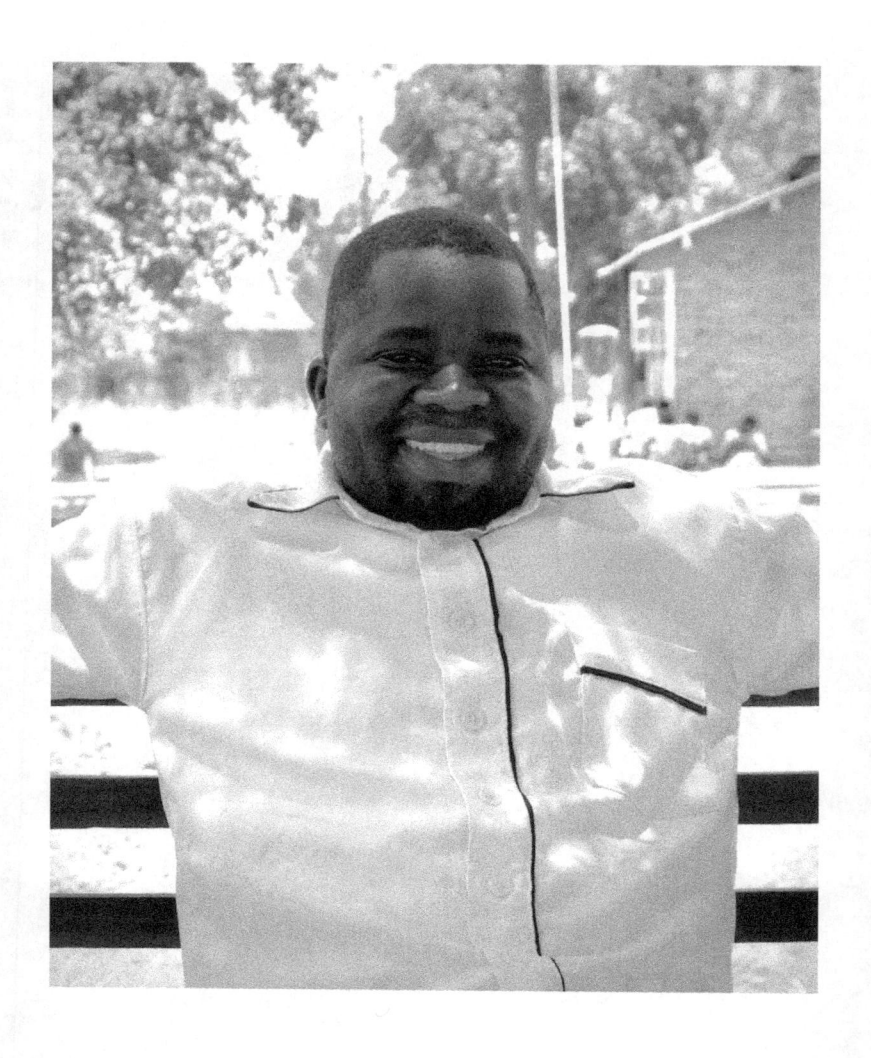

CHARLES #1 AND CHARLES #2

If there was one expectation that I had which was completely off, it was the amount of time—or lack thereof—that we spent at the Bimbi Health Facility. Going in, I had imagined that most of my days would be seeing the tall, brick walls of the facility, listening to the deep Chichewa voices murmuring behind the thin doors of the clinic. I pictured myself visiting the mothers and fathers at the clinic—a logical place of meeting if there ever was one. But in total, and I'm grateful for this, I must have sat on one of the open-air benches at the clinic a total of three times.

It was more effective and realistic that Agness took me to the doorstep of each of the people that I spoke with. In accordance with how the philosophies of the program works, the healing information and hope must be brought *to* the communities. Though I was ever grateful and appreciative of the off-white interior of the facility, I was pleased that my expectations were incorrect.

Making our way to the individual communities permitted an indulgence to my wide eyed and adventurous heart, landing me at the threshold of so many curious doorsteps. Beyond my own desires, taking the few extra steps to their individual homes allowed unquestionable insight to their life, setting and purpose for the maternal health program.

As it would seem, on this particular day our driver took us the familiar twists and turns on the dirt roads toward Bimbi, stopping the car in front of the facility. Agness and her team had a training course to administer to the nurses, and I was tagging along to speak with a few of them afterwards.

Agness and I had actually shown up late to the training, and the customary snack of Coca-Cola, orange Fanta, and sleeves of processed cookies were already being passed around. You couldn't go to any meeting or training event in Malawi where those few items weren't served. The trainees handed me a share and continued, discussing the best ways to include teenagers and young adults into the conversation of maternal health, family planning, and sexual health.

I listened to their passionate voices and honest tones, picking up the gist of their conversation through the speckled English terms and words that flowed seamlessly into their sentences. The school built right beside the facility had just been let out, and I distractedly gave myself over to the curious eyes and children's high voices—staring towards us as they followed the fence line along the road.

"*Mzungu!*" they called to me, running away in laughter when I waved.

Eventually the training concluded, and the nurses and Health Assistants waltzed back into their active lives—back to their homes or their shifts at the facility. I, on the other hand, pulled out my notebook and pen, ready for my part to begin.

I spoke with two men named Charles that afternoon. Charles #1 was an HSA and volunteer health worker in his village. He was in Bimbi for the training that had just concluded. Charles #2 was a nurse and midwife for the maternal ward in the facility. Both of them spoke English incredibly well, so Agness took her leave and caught up with her other nurses in the nearby shade, while I sat next to a broken bench and spoke with the two men.

"There was a lady in my village," Charles #1 began. "She was pregnant twice, but both of her children died. After the miscarriage of her second child, she also died. That's when I decided to work as an HSA."

"Wow," I took a breath in, still uncertain of the best way to respond to such heavy stories. "That's really honorable, Charles. Will you tell me some of the things that you do as an HSA?"

Charles #1 had small bones and a petite frame. There was a subtle tension in his posture, one that ran deeper than his nervous perch on the broken bench. I was grateful for the smile that gathered on the skin on his thin face, his eyes lit up in response.

"I encourage couples to come to the health facility in their first trimester of pregnancy."

I nodded, knowing there was a strong push for all expectant mothers to come in as soon as they could. The longer they have to monitor the mother and child, the more likely they are to be able to protect them from any complications that may arise.

"There is a problem of men never coming along to their partner's appointments," Charles #1 expanded. "It's important for men to be there—they have an impact on their families too!"

One of the major elements of Charles' work was to emphasize the importance of the father's participation in a family. When fathers come to their partner's appointments, it fosters a sense of responsibility, accountability, and involvement in the raising of their children. From there, couples are encouraged to think more carefully about family planning.

"Family planning," I repeated Charles' words back to him, scrawling furiously in my little blue notepad. "How would you define that?"

It was an important question, and it seemed to be the right one. Charles #1 was excited about this topic unlike any other.

"Family planning!" His eyes brightened, pulling his cheeks upwards. "I tell my community that it is a decision made by both the father and mother about how many children they want to have, and how many years in between."

Family planning is about making informed choices regarding sexual activities. An HSA or Health Promoter like Charles will go out and educate communities about cognizant sexual decisions and the importance of being intentional about their children. That includes providing information about contraceptives, child spacing, and eradicating inaccurate beliefs.

I was reading through a qualitative study recently conducted in regard to family planning in Malawi and was not surprised when I saw their results.

> "Overall, women were aware of both modern and traditional family planning methods, and the majority were in favour of modern versus

> traditional methods. They also had knowledge about risks for future complications if they have a short inter-pregnancy interval. However, they faced conflict about whether to use family planning methods for their health, as suggested by their relatives and friends, or to have another child to fulfil their husband's desire, especially among those with no living child. Some had fear about side effects, while others were concerned that use of family planning methods without involving the husband could bring misunderstandings within the family. A number of women had misconceptions about family planning methods, which also served as a barrier to their use." [xvii]

For me to understand, I had to mentally displace myself from the culture that I was raised in—where people thought about these things all the time. Since I was in eighth grade, my friends and I have been planning and dreaming about the families we may raise one day. I've chosen the names of my future children, I've decided how many I hope there to be, I've had a timeline in my mind for as long as I can remember. The ideas and dreams have fluctuated from time to time, changing as I do, but the reality is that I have never *not* participated in family planning. It took me a moment to acknowledge my North American culture in that matter before I understood— really understood—what Charles meant.

"Family planning actually helps develop Malawi. And not just our country, but it works internationally too. Before, there would be no time to develop the community!"

"What do you mean?"

"Well, things like building bridges, feeding rooms, constructing latrines... activities like that," Charles described. When parents establish more control over their family plans, they inevitably have more control over their time and resources. More control lends to greater impact, influence, and contribution to the overall community.

There were several mothers who assured me, "If I had known about family planning when I was younger, I would not have chosen to have so many children. But I didn't know that I had the choice."

Charles #2 was a handsome man. He was of a stockier build and carried a round face. All of the nurses, midwives, and HSAs were knowledgeable of and promoters of the same maternal health and healthier living material, but various elements tended to resonate differently between them. Charles #1 was passionate about family planning. Charles #2 had a heart to bring couples to the clinics and tend to them there.

"There's just so much more we can do for them at the clinic, we have more equipment here than they do at their homes!" he told me.

"Charles, can you explain something for me?"

He nodded. "Of course!"

"I'm just trying to understand. Why *wouldn't* women come to the facility when they're in labor? Why do they decide not to come?"

It was clear he often asked himself the same question. Charles shifted on the bench and smiled sadly. "Sometimes they won't come because there is no transportation and sometimes because they don't think they need to. I think it's a matter of ignorance—they just don't know. Or they think that they have the experience that they don't need to. They will say, 'No, this is my second, third, or fourth child. I already know what to do.'

"But if something happens..." He shifted again and brought his elbows to his knees, leaning forwards with a unique sense of urgency. "I would rather them be here at the facility so we can help."

The facility wasn't without its struggles either, however. Government programs and projects like PROMISE were doing the best they could to support and equip their facilities, but there were inevitably setbacks. Bimbi had a shortage of supplies. The nurses and midwives were often forced to make do with the equipment they had, but it wasn't always enough.

"We try our best. If there's any kind of complication, we call for transport to the nearest hospital. On a good day, we can get them there in two hours. On a bad day, you're looking at anywhere between twelve and fifteen hours."

By then, it's often too late.

Agness eventually made her way back to us and listened for a bit. Her head watched the light dust blowing on the ground, but her shoulders were set with a sense of pride. It was special for her to hear the passion and knowledge that her trainees spoke with and inspiring to hear their perspective.

Charles's final comment to me resonated true of all the people I had interacted with to date. It was profound in its simplicity, but an honest reflection of his heart.

"Sometimes I see mothers walking around and see they feel no relief. I say, let us help them!"

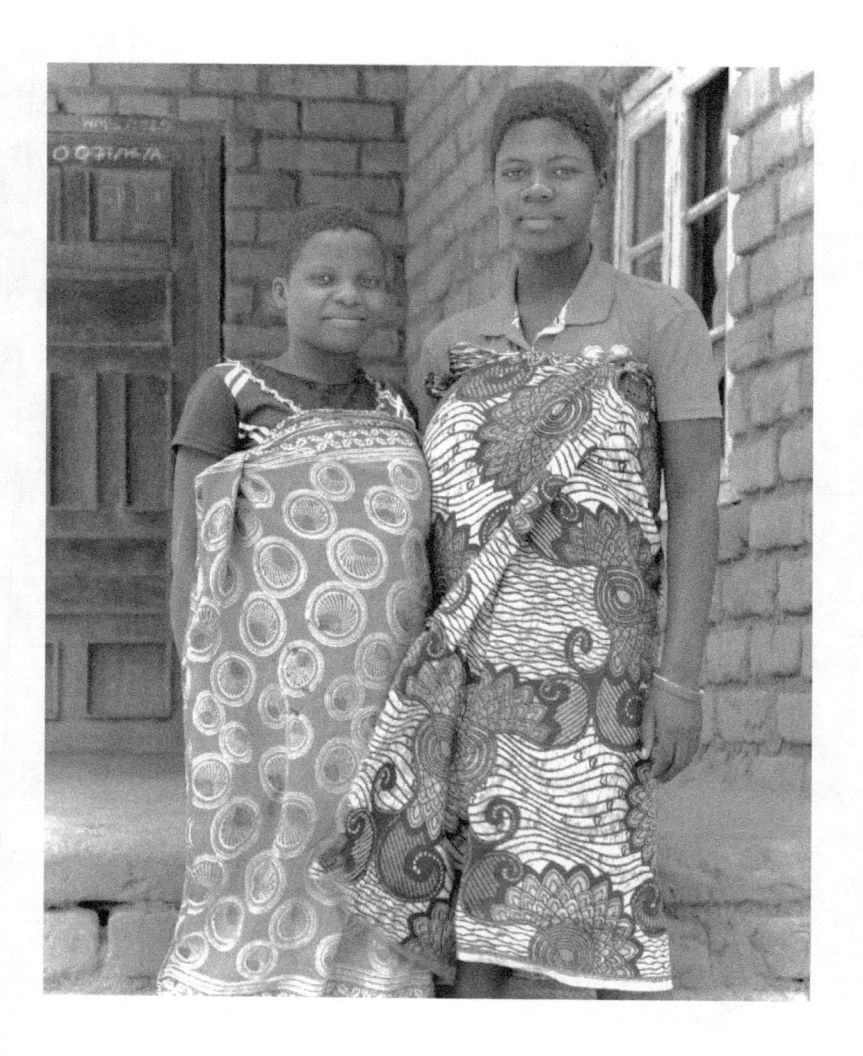

THE END

I don't know how to write this chapter.

You can see a thousand words in my notebook—written, crossed out, then written again. I'm still searching for the right combination of letters to adequately do justice to the powerful stories herein.

The weight of the subject is intimidating; in the depth of my love for the cause, today I faced the roots from which I've naïvely turned my eyes. Perhaps it's my optimistic mindset and trained resolve to focus on the good in a situation that has caused me to avoid this for so long. I've used it as coping mechanism to protect me from emotional cliffsides and darkened tunnels, but this distressing reality can be evaded no more.

It came unexpectedly, but this is perhaps the most important chapter in this book. I didn't know it would be like this, but I'm grateful it did, and I pray that you're listening.

Here's what I mean.

My last day in the field wasn't meant to be so impactful. Though I had three women to speak to, there were moments where I couldn't even formulate words. I asked Agness about it later on, and she agreed that she also hadn't anticipated their responses.

"It's a good reminder," she solemnly said. "This is why we're doing what we do. These women are the women who need Maternal Health more than anyone. They're exactly why we're out here."

"But how can it be like this?" I asked, not wanting to believe it—for their sake, and for the sake of nearly every woman in Malawi. For a second, I lost my hope. I saw the magnitude of the problem and wavered in the shadow of it. These three women and their stories are among the countless reasons for the mission of Maternal Health.

There was Miriam, Lydia, and Tinenengi. Agness had arranged to meet them with her contact in their village, explaining that we wanted to be introduced to expecting first-time mothers. I wanted to know about maternal health from their green perspective—their expectations of pregnancy, birth, and raising a child.

Up until this point, all of the men, women and children I had spoken with were those who could offer me a perspective of before and after maternal health programs had touched their lives. They were able to tell me, "This is what we endured before," with a smile because they could always follow it with, "This is how we live now."

It was always full of understanding, education, and hope.

But on this day, I tiptoed onto new ground that had not yet been touched by Maternal Health projects in Malawi.

Miriam, Lydia, and Tinenengi were all pregnant with their first children. Miriam and Tinenengi were eighteen; Lydia was seventeen. Two of the three pregnancies were unplanned, but as a result, all three of them were now married.

"I never expected to get pregnant," one of the women

explained to me. "I was in a relationship because my parents couldn't pay for my schooling. He would pay my school fees. But later I found out that I was pregnant, so now I don't go to school anyway."

I thought back to some of the mothers and nurses I had spoken to previously—how they told me that no education often led to early pregnancies, and vice-versa. It was a dangerous circle.

"I told my parents that I was pregnant, and they made us get married."

It was the same for the second mother, who told me her story. "We were neighbors. Neither of us were in school. When I discovered I was pregnant, both my parents and his parents agreed that we should be married."

I found it to be interesting that two of the three mothers-to-be had neither panned to get pregnant nor planned to be married. I wondered if it was an accurate ratio of planned versus unplanned pregnancy in their village, or if I had just stumbled into it by chance.

I wasn't shocked by this element of their story, however, and they didn't seem to share any disquiet over their stories either. I knew from much earlier that teenage pregnancy was correlated to education (or lack thereof) and the consequences that an unexpected child could bring to the mother.

No, it wasn't their unplanned pregnancies or marriages or nonchalant way they spoke about them that moved me to speechlessness. It was the fact that all three of them collectively had no idea what to expect.

"So, how is it going?" I asked them. "Is being pregnant anything like you thought it would be?"

I watch Agness squirm, playing with the dirt that had hardened into stone as she listened to their answers.

"I can't really see the difference between now and what I expected," Agness crumbled the dirt between her fingers. "Because I had never really heard about pregnancies before."

"I was once told about the signs of labor," said one of the young women. "So, I suppose I'll know when the time comes."

"You're right," the first responded. "And I once heard I should be breastfeeding my child once they come. And feeding them!"

Miriam, the one who planned her pregnancy, offered similar thoughts. "From what I have been explained, I think it's just about eating a balanced diet. Then my baby will be fine."

I thought about what Charles had told me the day prior. *It's a matter of ignorance. They just don't know.*

Though aware of it, I was unprepared to see the depth of that honest ignorance, and how it sharply contrasted the knowledge that mothers who had been part of a maternal health program now had.

Neither Miriam, Lydia, nor Tinnenegi were to blame for their ignorance. Their mothers and grandmothers weren't to blame either. These mamas, their future little ones, and all of Malawi that they represent are innocent victims to the nature of the culture of poor maternal health. They walk the same path that teeters on the ledge of the cliff as they have always done, not knowing of the safer trail lying just beside it.

"But have you thought at all about what you'll do when you have your child?" I asked. "What are your plans?"

I waited patiently for the round of translation to make its way back to me. I watched as Miriam's head made a curious tilt, and she responded passively. "No... I haven't thought about what I will do. I think I will just plan later."

"But what about the clinic? Have you been to a clinic for any check-ups?" I was pleading now, begging that she would say yes. She was in her sixth month of pregnancy—surely, she had seen at least one nurse.

But her answer was negative and non-committal, "No. Maybe I'll go sometime this week."

On some occasions, Agness would continue speaking to the women or men that we were engaging with, often clarifying what my questions were, or asking questions of her own. I loved her for it, known she was just as invested in the conversation as I was. But I could tell that Agness was unsettled by these three stories, taking more time than usual with their Chichewa clarification.

It was a long drive home. We drove about an hour farther into the horizon, through snaking roads that alone I could have never found my way out of. We sent clouds of dust blooming behind us as our white truck bounced over the untamed potholes and ruts. I resigned my worries of being lost to the expertise of our driver and turned my attention to the complete consumption and memorization of the landscape.

We inched our way over a broken land-bridge that interrupted a large, empty floodplain. Mountains were in the hazy distance, and I soaked it all in. I have no photograph but the savory picture in my mind's eye to relive it. The beauty is a memory tucked away in a treasured place in my mind.

We ended up in the courtyard of a school where the

rest of the Maternal Health team had delivered a training on nutrition. Remaining with them for the final touches of their data collection, we only set out on the long road back when the rest of the team was ready to return with us.

By the time we made it to home base, we were watching the last breath of sunshine softly sink beneath the mountains.

"Are you afraid?" I asked Miriam earlier that day.

Her answer has rung in my ears ever since I heard it.

It has been the inspiration to the many chapters of this book, echoing silently throughout the pages. Her answer, simple, quiet and unknowingly profound has been my personal propeller as I relay the testimonies within.

Her answer is the resounding reason that Maternal Health is so imperative to promote.

"Are you afraid?" I asked the eighteen-year-old mother-to-be sitting timidly on the Malawian dirt.

Agness paused before she translated.

"People tell me that I should be afraid. They tell me I might die. But I tell them to wait and see what happens."

WORKS CITED

[i] "Maternal Mortality." World Health Organization, World Health Organization, 19 Sept. 2019, www.who.int/en/news-room/fact-sheets/detail/maternal-mortality.

[ii] "Millennium Development Goals (MDGs)." World Health Organization, World Health Organization, 19 Feb. 2018, www.who.int/topics/millennium_development_goals/en/.

[iii] Republic of Malawi. "About Us." The Ministry of Health and Population, 2018. www.health.gov.mw/index.php/explore/management.

[iv] Boerma, Ties, and Carine Ronsmans, et al. "Global Epidemiology of Use of and Disparities in Caesarean Sections." *The Lancet*, vol. 394, no. 10192, 2019, p. 25.

[v] "Maternal and Newborn Health Disparities Country Profiles-Malawi." UNICEF DATA, 25 Sept. 2018, data.unicef.org/resources/maternal-newborn-health-disparities-country-profiles/.

[vi] "Maternal, Neonatal, and Child Health: Malawi." U.S. Agency for International Development, 15 Nov. 2019, www.usaid.gov/malawi/global-health/maternal-neonatal-and-child-health.

[vii] Mothe, Anke. Personal Interview. October 2018.

[viii] International Food Policy Research Institute (IFPRI). "Agriculture, Food Security, and Nutrition in Malawi: Leveraging the Links," 2018.

[ix] Egholm, D.L., et al. "The Mechanics of Clay Smearing along Faults." Geology, vol. 36, no. 10, 2008, p. 787.

[x] Disabled World. "Average Height to Weight Chart: Babies to Teenagers." Disabled World, Disabled World, 7 Oct. 2020, www.disabled-world.com/calculators-charts/height-weight-teens.php.

[xi] "Malawi: Nutrition Profile." U.S. Agency for International Development, 11 Sept. 2019, www.usaid.gov/global-health/health-areas/nutrition/countries/malawi-nutrition-profile.

[xii] Ibid

[xiii] "Maternal and Newborn Health Disparities Country Profiles." UNICEF DATA, 25 Sept. 2018, data.unicef.org/resources/maternal-newborn-health-disparities-country-profiles/.

[xiv] "Malawi Infant Mortality Rate." World Data Atlas, Knoema, 2019. knoema.com/atlas/Malawi/Infant-mortality-rate.

[xv] "Gender Equality and Women's Empowerment: Malawi." U.S. Agency for International Development, 15 Nov. 2019, www.usaid.gov/gender-equality-and-womens-empowerment.

[xvi] "Malawi Gender Equality Fact Sheet." U.S. Agency for International Development, USAID, 26 Sept. 2016, www.usaid.gov/malawi/fact-sheets/malawi-gender-equality-fact-sheet.

[xvii] Bula, Agatha, et al. "Family Planning Knowledge, Experiences and Reproductive Desires among Women Who Had Experienced a Poor Obstetric Outcome in Lilongwe Malawi: A Qualitative Study." *Contraception and Reproductive Medicine*, BioMed Central, 17 Oct. 2018, www.ncbi.nlm.nih.gov/pmc/articles/PMC6192333/.

Additional Resources:

"Malawi GDP per capita 1960–2019 Data: 2020–2021 Forecast: Historical: Chart." Malawi GDP per Capita Chart, tradingeconomics.com/malawi/gdp-per-capita.

Nutrition Handbook for Farmer Field Schools. May 2015, www.fao.org/fileadmin/user_upload/nutrition/docs/education/resources/by_country/Malawi/FFS_Nutrition_Handbook.pdf.

UNICEF. Nutrition Statistics in Malawi, MalawiUNICEF, 2018.
CCFC Ghana, et al. 2018, PROMISE Midterm Survey Report.
CCFC Ghana, et al. March 2017, PROMISE Annual Report – Year 2.
CCFC Ghana, et al. June 2018, PROMISE

ACKNOWLEDGEMENTS

The first song of praise must always go to God, whose faithfulness shines so clearly in the orchestration of this book and its contents. In the days where my confidence and faith faltered, His purpose prevailed. To the individuals their families mentioned in this book, thank you for your honesty, your openness, and perseverance. Your stories have the capacity to change the world; *Zikomo*.

To my handsome husband, thank you for your endless examples of perseverance, consistency, and strength. To my parents and brothers, thank you for supporting my journey and not protesting too much when I insist on leaping headfirst into new adventures. To Paul and Helen Jones, who have opened their doors to countless missionaries and workers, thank you for your massive contribution to these stories. You inspire me towards a more selfless life. To EIC, ADRA, and Children Believe, your maternal health efforts through PROMISE have sent a beacon of light to a world that so desperately needed it. Thank you.

Finally, thank you to Bridgehead Coffee in Ottawa, who fueled my 6:00 am writing habits and fulfilled my lifelong dream of becoming a recognized coffee-shop regular.

ABOUT THE AUTHOR

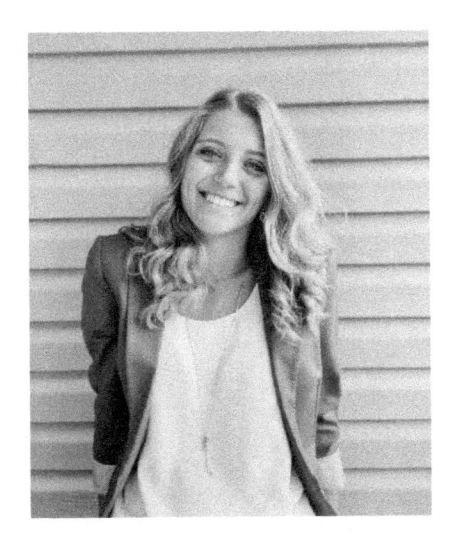

Canadian author Caitlin Arlene is known for her love of strangers and their stories. Her short works have been published in various periodicals such as the *Toronto Star*, *Christianity Today*, and the *Ottawa Citizen*. Migrating throughout Ontario with her husband, who serves as an Officer in the Canadian Armed Forces, Caitlin Arlene spends her free time basking in the sunshine and hunting down local coffee shops.

ABOUT ATMOSPHERE PRESS

Atmosphere Press is an independent, full-service publisher for excellent books in all genres and for all audiences. Learn more about what we do at atmospherepress.com.

We encourage you to check out some of Atmosphere's latest releases, which are available at Amazon.com and via order from your local bookstore:

Out and Back: Essays on a Family in Motion, by Elizabeth Templeman
Just Be Honest, by Cindy Yates
You Crazy Vegan: Coming Out as a Vegan Intuitive, by Jessica Ang
Detour: Lose Your Way, Find Your Path, by S. Mariah Rose
To B&B or Not to B&B: Deromanticizing the Dream, by Sue Marko
Convergence: The Interconnection of Extraordinary Experiences, by Barbara Mango and Lynn Miller
Sacred Fool, by Nathan Dean Talamantez
My Place in the Spiral, by Rebecca Beardsall
My Eight Dads, by Mark Kirby
Dinner's Ready! Recipes for Working Moms, by Rebecca Cailor
Vespers' Lament: Essays Culture Critique, Future Suffering, and Christian Salvation, by Brian Howard Luce